YOGIC CURE
TO
AVOID HEART SURGERY

YOGIC CURE
TO
AVOID HEART SURGERY

> Treatment of Coronary Heart Disease through Yoga:
> Exercises, Asanas, Pranayama, Kayotsarga, Meditation,
> Stress Management, Diet Management, and Yogic Life-Style

Author
Dr B. L. JAIN
M.Sc., Ph.D.

Technical Adviser
Dr J. P. N. MISHRA
M. Sc., Ph. D.

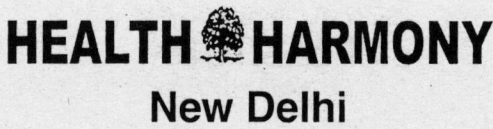

HEALTH HARMONY
New Delhi

> *Note:*
>
> Any information given in this book is not intended to be taken as a replacement for medical advice. Any person with a condition requiring medical attention should consult a qualified practitioner or therapist.

Reprint Edition: 2006
First revised edition : 2001

All rights are reserved. No part of this publication may be reproduced, stored in a retrieval system or transmitted in any form or by any means mechanical recording or otherwise without prior written permission of the publishers.

Price: Rs: 199.00

© Copyright Reserved

Published by :
Kuldeep Jain
for

HEALTH ❦ HARMONY

an imprint of
B. Jain Publishers (P) Ltd.
1921 Street No.10 Chuna Mandi,
Paharganj, New Delhi 110 055 (INDIA)
Phones: 91-011-2358 0800, 2358 1100, 2358 1300
Fax: 91-011-2358 0471; Email: bjain@vsnl.com
Website: www.bjainbooks.com

Printed in India by:
Unisons Techno Financial Consultants (P) Ltd.
522, FIE, Patpar Ganj, Delhi 110 092

ISBN: 81-8056-004-X
Book Code: BJ-5561

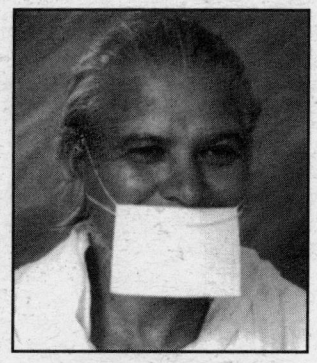

Acharya Shiv Muni

Dated: September 18th, 2001

BLESSINGS

Good health is the optimum physiological functioning physical as well as mental. A healthy mind stays only in a healthy body. Our body gets a disease due to several internal and external reasons, which ultimately causes hindrance in our worldly and spiritual activities.

Heart diseases are the prominent ones among several others that make both body and mind sick. The only way to prosperous, disease free, joyous, with peaceful mind and body, is to adopt Yogic Life Style.

This is equally applicable in the state of abnormal heart functioning. I believe that Yoga and Meditation therapy suggested by the author of this book will be of great help to the patients of heart disease.

I send my blessings for the success of this endeavour.

(ACHARYA SHIV MUNI)
Head: All India Shwetambar Jain Sthanak Vasi Shraman Sangh.

DEDICATED

TO

MY WIFE

LATE JAIN VATI JAIN

who was

MY SPIRITUAL INSPIRER

FOREWORD

Coronary heart disease (CHD) nowadays has become the largest killer in developed countries and is rapidly assuming a similar role among the middle and upper income group people in India too.

Stress is a global phenomenon and is the main causative factor of CHD. Today it has become an inevitable companion in all walks of life. Biological stress always remains with us in one form or the other from birth to death. One cannot avoid it. It has to be managed.

The twenty-first century may show an unprecedented rise in the incidence of stress-related diseases, like coronary heart disease, if we do not adopt proper measures of stress management. This is the focal theme of this presentation.

Yoga has prophylactic, promotive and curative potential. These basic techniques of yoga and preksha meditation are well elaborated in this book. It will be quite convenient to understand the step-by-step process of yogasanas, pranayama and meditation, as methodological aspects have been presented very lucidly here and in a simple manner. Stress-management techniques and various tips related to the management of CHD are also described lucidly.

Another important facet of this book is the compilation of yogic life-style and diet-style principles, which may prove very helpful in managing CHD.

Apart from the theoretical explanations of CHD, its pathological discription and causative factors along with the probable therapeutic role of yoga and meditation, supportive data from the experimental studies carried out on CHD patients by the author, make the book an invaluable practical guide for managing CHD.

Realising the need to inform the common people of our society about the fundamentals and also to provide composite information about coronary heart disease and its management through yoga, this noble task has been undertaken by a well qualified, experienced and dedicated author in a very simple, practical, scientific and effective manner in this book. I am confident that the sojourn through the book can convince the readers as well as CHD patients to change their life-styles and ameliorate stress reaction by providing a positive attitude and sound health to manage as well as prevent CHD.

Dr. J. P. N. Mishra
Head
Dep. of Science of Living,
Preksha Meditation & Yoga,
Jain Vishwa Bharati Institute,
Ladnun (Rajasthan)

Yogic Cure to Avoid Heart Surgery

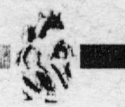

Dr Abdul Aziz
M.B.B.S., M.S.
Ex Chief Medical Officer
Delhi Vidyut Board
New Delhi

During the contemporary times of materialistic, highly competitive and extremely ambitious life-style, to which the human being is exposed, the human body, mind and soul is subjected to tremendous autonomous and hormonal stresses and strains. They lead to diseases such as essential hypertension, coronary artery or heart disease, diabetes mellitus, bronchial asthama and mental disorders, and a large number of collagen diseases like psoriasis, polyarthritis etc. have become a common occurance, to which no curative remedy is available even in today's modern system of medicines. Whatever is being done in the form of transplants, graft and plasty surgeries and other high-tech, costly mode of treatment, is only palliative in nature that require life-long medication to maintain the quality of life after each such procedure.

Of late it is now being realized even by specialists in modern medicine that meditation, transcendental meditation and yogic exercises/asanas greatly reduce the stresses and strains from the autonomous system and neuro-endocrine system of human body, which in turn help reduce the incidence or the intensity of above mentioned chronic and incurable diseases. In addition, the practice of meditation and yogic exercises/asanas is not only free of financial involvement but also require only a few minutes of regularity each day. Obviously, there is no question of any medication in such practices.

Dr B. L. Jain has very successfully brought home the mesage to the general public not conversant with the medical terminology and knowledge as such, that by sparing a fraction of time daily, they can tone up their body, mind and soul to ward off such incurable diseases like hypertention and coronary heart disease without any medication, monetary expenditure or side effects.

I wish Dr B.L. Jain every success in this pioneering effort and cause.

New Delhi
15 January 2001

Dr Abdul Aziz

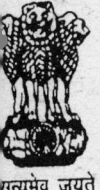

डा0 अशोक कुमार वालिया
DR. ASHOK KUMAR WALIA

स्वास्थ्य, शहरी विकास, पर्यावरण, वन, वन्य जीव एवं चुनाव मंत्री
MINISTER OF HEALTH, URBAN DEVELOPMENT, ENVIRONMENT,
FOREST, WILD LIFE AND ELECTION
राष्ट्रीय राजधानी क्षेत्र दिल्ली सरकार
GOVT OF NATIONAL CAPITAL TERRITORY OF DELHI
दिल्ली सचिवालय, आई० पी० एस्टेट, नई दिल्ली-110002
DELHI SECRETARIATE, IP. ESTATE, NEW DELHI-110002
TEL. NO :
D O. No. MIM/20../4662
दिनांक /

Dated :   22 December 2000

MESSAGE

    I am glad to learn that Dr B. L. Jain, M. Sc., Ph. D. has attempted a book entitled "Yogic Cure to Avoid Heart Surgery".

    It is a well-known fact that, of late, the number of patients of coronary heart disease is on the rise all over the world. Although there are many causes of heart ailments like improper diet, lack of physical exercise, ignorance of health rules etc., but to my mind, stress is one of the main reasons for prevalence of this disease. Biological stress is the one that cannot be avoided. It has just to be managed. Dr B. L. Jain in his book has focused on treatment of coronary heart disease (CHD) by Yogasana, Pranayama and Meditation instead of painful surgery or life-long medication.

    I hope the book will provide composite information to the readers about CHD and its management through yoga, which will be beneficial for the heart patients in particular and the masses in general. Dr Jain deserves commendation for putting in all out efforts in bringing out this useful book. I wish him all success in life.

(DR A. K. WALIA)

PREFACE

Man is the most beautiful creation of God upon earth. The heart, fitted in the human body and functioning there, is a piece of great miracle. It beats rhythmically with unfailing regularity and looks after the requirment of every organ, every tissue and every cell. Man is compelled to admit the power of the Creater for creating this marvellous wonder, but he has always been under-assessing its worth and has not taken proper care of this vital organ.

The man, by nature, wants to remain healthy, wealthy and happy. In the modern age of tension, pollution, dependence on science and mechanical life-style, not only in India but throughout the world, people are running after money with closed eyes. They do not care for their morals, principles, duty towards self or nation. Man is ready to sell himself, his body, his mind and even his country for money.

The government has opened various schools, colleges, education centres and universities to educate the people in this regard. In India, yogis and spiritual preachers are trying to communicate the actual meaning of education but the results are not very satisfying. No system of education is effective in inculcating eternal values till it is connected, directly or indirectly, with earning of money nowadays.

In modern age the needs have overpowered man in such a way that people of all classes and categories find themselves incapable of coping up with the varied and ever-mounting materialistic demands and requirements. All this causes big stress in the individuals of the society.

As a result, the people have become dishonest, fearful, unhealthy, violent, greedy and drug addicts, lacking physical activities, tolerance, truthfulness and contentment, which brings them to a stressful state, thus creating psychosomatic diseases, viz. diabetes, hypertension, acidity, peptic ulcers, cervical spondylosis and, above all, blockage in arteries that leads to cornonary heart disease (CHD).

This situation has brought the whole world on a point of no return and man now finds himself helpless. Man today is running fearfully towards an unknown imaginary goal.

In view of the existing circumstances, the present remedial medical treatments for coronary heart disease have become insufficient in providing adequate cure of the disease. At times the present therapy's results are unfavourable. As a matter of fact the so-called modern therapies are not treating or curing the disease but are rather maintaining it. Neither do they let the patient die nor do they let him/her be cured. They help the patient to continue surviving, but with the disease, so that the consumption of medicines is increased and the pharmaceutical industries flourish.

The health of man is basically of a psychosomatic nature and the modern therapies are treating only the somatic part, whereas the yoga, since ancient times is treating the diseases psychosomatically. But with the passage of time, yoga was suppressed, ignored and discontinued, perhaps because India remained under foreign subjugation for centuries together. Yogic practices aim to strengthen the heart and whole body, enabling them to get rid of the disease. Now is the right time for taking yoga therapy into account for treating CHD.

HOW DID THE IDEA OF WRITING THIS BOOK COME ?

The idea of writing this book came just as a lightning flash. When I was doing my M.Sc. in Science of Living and Preksha Meditation (Yoga), I found that various somatic and psychosomatic diseases were curable through yoga. I then thought why CHD could not be cured by yoga? Why people spend lakhs of rupees for bypass/ open-heart surgery and take risks? I then started to concentrate my studies towards methods of yoga for treating coronary heart disease and studied it deeply.

In the mean time, unfortunately, one of my close relatives suffered from coronary heart disease. He was taking treatment in a government hospital. They were giving him proper allopathic medicines such as Sorbitrate, Monotrate and Disprin.

The patient was happy and was following doctor's advice and precautions. He was doing well. Whenever he used to feel chest pain, they used to add a tablet or two every time. Gradually the number of tablets reached 30 a day, but the disease was not cured or lessened. At last he was advised bypass surgery. He got it done but the pain and medicines continued. The doctors were not able to justify the purpose of bypass surgery performed on him.

Days passed and the quantity of medicines also increased. His chest pain was never cured and one fine morning we learnt that the patient had left this world forever. Perhaps this happens in most of the CHD cases. I was shaken when I learnt

Preface

about the sad demise of my dear one and was compelled to think over why the patient was not cured when he was so well-to-do and financially sound to bear the treatment cost, and was following all the precautions and advices of the doctor. At last I reached the conclusion that the modern medicines are actually not treating or curing the disease but are only maintaining the state of the disease. They never try to go deep to find the root cause of the disease to eliminate it. The disease does not leave the patient, but the patient leaves the world.

The idea struck that the CHD could be treated through yoga, and immediately I started working on the topic.

The book in your hands is the outcome of this project. It deals with eradication of the disease through removal of stress by delving into the root of the problem with proper explanation of the cause and cure of coronary heart disease, by adopting the 'Innovative Yogic Life-style Intervention Programme'. I hope it will help people to lead a happy and healthy life.

Dr B. L. Jain

CAUTION

*Y*ogic exrsises and asanas peracited without expert guidence and proper caution, may harm you. Therefore better consult your doctor before taking up this or any exercise programme. The advice, instructions and exercises suggested in this programme are in no way intended as a substitute for medical counselling. Continue with your regular medication, begin slowly the yogic exercises etc. suggested in this book as a supplementary cure, gradually increasing their duration and intensity while having regular check-up with your physician/doctor following that advice faithfully, especially for any anatomical, physiological or serious disorder. The programme suggested in the book would gradually tone up your body and add strength to the muscles and organs to fight back the disease.

ACKNOWLEDGEMENTS

First, I am thankful to the Almighty God who has helped me a lot at each stage of my work and enabled me to complete the book in time.

The presentation would not be complete without expressing my deep gratitute towards all those who supported me in this work. First, I owe my most sincere thanks to my friend and consultant Dr J.P.N. Mishra, Head, Department of Science of Living and Preksha Meditation, Jain Vishwa Bharati Institute (Deemed University), Ladnun (Rajasthan), who has always encouraged me to complete the task specially during the moments I was tense and losing interest in the work. He not only helped me in preparing the manuscript, but also contributed academically as if he himself was writing this book.

I shall be failing in my duty if I do not express my gratitude to Dr Bimal Chhajer, MD, Managing Director, Saaol Health (P) Ltd, New Delhi. He is the gentleman who actually lighted the flame in me and inspired me to start the work.

A gesture of gratitude towards my friends and family members especially my son, Anil Jain, who has always been inspiring/ encouraging me not only in person but also telepathically to make the project a success. My appreciation is also extended to my wife Mrs J.V. Jain and my daughter in law Mrs Kusum Jain for their esteemed co-operation and help.

My special thanks to Swami Dharmanandji, Director, Adhyatm Sadhana Kendra, Mehrauli, New Delhi, Dr J.S. Raghuvanshi, Chairman, Centre for Research in Alternative System of Medicines and International Brotherhood, East Patel Nagar, New Delhi; Shri N.P. Gang, Director, Jivan Vigyan Academy, and Shri Madan Kumar Jain, Director, Tulsi Adhyatm Needam, Ladnun for their valuable guidance and arranging interviews with patients attending their centres. I am also thankful to my subjects for their relevant valuable questions stimulating me to write this book and their families, without whose co-operation this work would not have been accomplished.

Lastly, my special thanks to my best friends Dr Abdul Aziz, Dr V.K. Bindal, Dr Asha Baluja, Dr V.P Jain, Dr V.D. Sharma, Dr S.K. Jain, Dr Santosh Jain, Mr Lajpat Rai Jain, Mr. & Mrs. Sanjeev Dhir, Mr J.P. Kaushal and Mr Piyush Sharma for their valuable academic help. Finally, I feel indebted to the publishers - Mr P. N. Jain, Mr Kuldeep Jain, Mr. Sarwan Jain and Mr. Rahul Sharma for offering their perceptive and extremely helpful response at various stages of preparation of the manuscript and taking keen interest in publishing this work.

I once again pay my thanks to everyone who assisted and co-operated with me in any way during the entire period of planning and publishing this work.

Dr B. L. JAIN
Author

CONTENTS

Foreword	vii
Preface	xii
Acknowledgements	xv

INTRODUCTION — 1
Section 1 : Human Body and Heart — 5

Chapter 1 : Know Your Body — 7

1.1	Human machine	9
1.2	Cell	10
1.3	Organs system	10
1.4	Skeletal system	10
1.5	Muscular system	11
1.6	Integumentary system (Skin)	11
1.7	Digestive system	11
1.8	Circulatory system	11
1.9	Respiratory system	12
1.10	Excretory system	13
1.11	Nervous system	13
1.12	Sense organs	13
1.13	Endocrine system	14
1.14	Reproductive system	14

Chapter 2 : Know Your Heart — 15

2.1	Introduction	17
2.2	Structure of heart	17
2.3	Heart : miracle pump	17
2.4	Blood circulation	18
2.5	Four heart chambers	19
2.6	Four major heart valves	20
2.7	Blood vessels — arteries, capillaries	21

2.8	Pulmonary veins and arteries	21
2.9	Aorta	22
2.10	Nourishment of heart and coronary arteries	22
2.11	Cardiac output	22
2.12	Blood stream and composition of blood	23
2.13	Heart beat and pulse	23

Chapter 3 : Cardiac Problems — 25

3.1	Angina	27
3.2	Heart attack	27
3.3	How to recognise angina and heart attack	28
3.4	Hypertension (high blood pressure)	28
3.5	Systolic and diastolic pressure	28
3.6	Prevention of heart attack, angina and hypertension	28

➤ Yogic life-style, diet control, regular physical exercise, avoid mental tension, stop smoking, regular medical check-up

Section 2 : Coronary Heart Disease — 31

Chapter 4 : Coronary Heart Disease — 33

4.1	Introduction	35
4.2	Coronary thrombosis	35
4.3	Conventional management of CHD	36
4.4	Medical management	36

➤ Vasodilators, anti-platelet drugs, drugs that reduce oxygen demand of heart

4.5	Surgical management	37

➤ Pace-maker, angioplasty, bypass surgery (open-heart surgery)

Chapter 5 : Diagnostic Techniques for Coronary Heart Disease — 41

5.1	Common diagnostic devices	43
5.2	ECG (Electrocardiogram)	43
5.3	Blood test (lipid profile test)	43
5.4	Echocardiography (Ultrasound Scan)	44
5.5	T.M.T. (Stress test)	44
5.6	Thallium scan	45
5.7	Pet scan	45
5.8	Angiography	45
5.9	Possible drawbacks and complications of angiography	45

	5.10	Commercialisation of angiography	46
	5.11	Other chest pains and angina	46
	➤	Muscular chest pain, cervical pain in left or right arm, gastric pain in chest	

Chapter 6 :   **Causative Factors of Coronary Heart Disease**   **47**

	6.1	Introduction	49
	6.2	Non-modifiable risk factors	50
	➤	Age, sex, heredity	
	6.3	Modifiable risk factors	50
	➤	Irregular life-style, stress and mental tension, lack of physical activity, faulty dietary habits, high blood pressure, notorious cholesterol, high blood-cholesterol level, high blood-triglyceride level, high blood-LDL and VLDL levels, high density lipoprotien (HDL) level, diabetes mellitus, obesity, lack of anti-oxidants in diet, isolation, hostility, self-centredness, cynicism, job stress, family stress, greed, sedentary life, smoking and alcohol	

Section 3 : Stress and Coronary Heart Disease   59

Chapter 7 :   **Stress**   **61**

	7.1	Introduction	63
	7.2	What is stress?	63
	7.3	Salient factors of overload stress	64
	➤	Work overload, time overload, requirement overload, information overload, sickness overload	
	7.4	Seven sectors of life synthesis	67
	➤	Work and profession, money, health, family, love and affection, social life, spiritual atmosphere	
	7.5	Stress and psychosomatic diseases	68
	7.6	Salient symptoms of excessive stress	69
	➤	Physical symptoms, behavioural symptoms, emotional symptoms, cognitive symptoms, physiological symptoms	

Chapter 8 :		Stress Management	71
	8.1	Introduction	73
	8.2	Ideal stress	73
	8.3	Excessive stress	73
	8.4	Production of stress	73
	➢	Internal stressers, external stressers, environmental stressers	
	8.5	Keys to cope with stress	74
	➢	Recognition and identification of stress, avoiding and forgetting the incidences, minor modification in routine matters to cope with stress	
	8.6	Strategies for stress management	75
	➢	When you are angry, when anger has cooled down but chronic stress of anger is present, skill of communication, anuvrat (development of moral values), anekant (theory of multiple views or non-absolutism), anupreksha (development of will power)	
	8.7	Skill of time management	77
	8.8	Jotting down exercises	78
	8.9	Meditation	79
	8.10	Kayotsarga (self-relaxation)	79

Section 4 : Yogic Management of Coronary Heart Disease   81

Chapter 9 :		Yoga as a Remedy for Inadequate Modern Drugs in CHD	83
	9.1	Introduction	85
	9.2	Symposium on problems of drug resistance in different diseases	85
	9.3	National conference of yoga reasearch and application	86

Chapter 10 :		Yoga: Concept, Components and Therapy	89
	10.1	Introduction	91
	10.2	Basis of yoga therapy	91
	10.3	Yoga fundamentals	92
	10.4	Patanjali's yoga sutra (ashtang yoga)	94
	➢	Yama, niyama, asanas, pranayama, pratyahara, dharana, dhyana, samadhi	
	10.5	Preksha yoga (seven steps)	99
	➢	Kayotsarga, antaryatra, shwas preksha, sharir preksha, chaitanya	

kendra preksha, leshya dhyana, therapeutic thinking through auto-suggestion and contemplation
    10.6 Benefits of preksha yoga   103
    10.7 Benefits of kayotsarga   103
    ➢ Relief from tension, freedom from turmoil, revitalisation of the organism, self-awareness, development of aura, development of wisdom

Chapter 11 :   **Yogic Management of Coronary Heart Disease in India and Abroad**   **107**

    11.1 Dean Ornish's concept of CHD reversal through yoga   109
    11.2 Treatment of CHD through yoga in India   110

Section 5 : Dietary Management   111

Chapter 12 :   **Dietary Management**   **113**

    12.1 Role of diet in managing CHD   115
    12.2 Nutrients   116
    12.3 CHD reversal diet   117
    12.4 Anti-oxidants of food   117
    12.5 An ideal food chart for CHD patients   118
    ➢ Breakfast, lunch, evening tea, dinner
    12.6 How to prepare zero-oil food   119
    12.7 Food items   121
    ➢ Restricted, moderately restricted, freely consumable

Section 6 : An Innovative Yogic Life-style Intervention Programme   123

Chapter 13 :   **Innovative Yogic Life-style Intervention Programme for CHD Management**   **125**

    13.1 Introduction   127
    13.2 Components of the programme   127
    ➢ Health-rejuvenating yogic exercises: 128
(head and mind, eyes, neck, ears, face, shoulders, chest and lungs, waist, thighs and hips, feet, knees, ankles, toes and heels), kayotsarga
    ➢ Yogic asanas   136
(Tadasana, Padahastasana, Vajrasana, Sashankasana, Ardhchan-

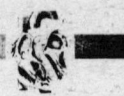

    drasana, Ardhamatsyendrasana, Uttanpadasana, Merudandasana, Bhujangasana, Shalabhasana, Pawanmuktasana)
- General conditions for performing asanas
- Benefits of asnas
- Precautions for asanas
- Pranayama (breathing exercise):   143
  abdominal breathing, anulom-vilom pramayama, om dhwani and laughter
- Benefits of pranayama
- Precautions for pranayama
- Mudras: 146
  (apan mudra, vyan mudra)
- Kayotsarga (total relaxation with self-awareness)   147
- Preksha Meditation (special meditation for CHD patients)   148

Chapter 14 :   **Efficacy of Yogic Life-style Intervention Programme in Reversing/ Managing CHD (Experimental Research Results)**   **151**

 14.1 Introduction   153
 14.2 Comparative data of CHD patients   153
   (before and after yoga therapy)
 14.3 Discussion and conclusions   160

Annexures: 161

1. Height-and-weight chart for adults (men/women)   163
2. Contents of nutrients in some common food items   164
3. Seven golden rules for CHD prevention   165
4. Cardio - pulmonary resuscitation (CPR)   166
5. Standard daily routine chart for CHD patients   169
6. Special benefits of exercises/asanas and pranayama   170
7. Special benefits of meditation and kayotsarga   170
8. Emergency Stress Releasing kit   171
9. Some clarifications sought by various CHD patients   172
10. Useful instructions for CHD patients   173

INTRODUCTION

Our state of health reflects an integration of all functions of our life. These include physical, mental, emotional, social and spiritual aspects. The main problem is that the way of our living, our life style that is vital to our health, is full of faults, which ultimately leads to various systemic diseases and disorders. As described by World Health Organisation, health is a state of complete physical, mental and social well-being and not merely the absence of disease and infirmity. The term "State of well-being" itself depends upon the manner we lead our daily life. The practice of health care in the so called advanced and modern system of living implies that our understanding of health is very unintegrated.

Significant advances in the medical science over the past century have reduced the incidence of most of the physical diseases that have plagued humanity for centuries. Better drugs and surgical techniques have led to the eradication of most infectious diseases and control of many metabolic disorders. But these techniques are less effective against the new and even more common causes of ill health—chronic stress and psychosomatic ailments. Coronary heart disease is one such disease that is causing great concern because of its fast spread among the various strata of society.

Conventional medicine, by concentrating on a physical and mechanical approach to healing, can do little to relieve such abnormal pathological states, since these are caused more by life-style and attitudes than by physiological abnormalities. The fast-moving and mechanical life exposes many people to continuous, unrelieved stress. And if a person is largely sedentary in his or her habits and overindulgent in health-damaging substances and foods, his/her well-being and fitness will be further compromised. Coronary heart disease (CHD) is a fast-spreading pathological state in human-beings from all sectors of the society and in this century it is going to assume an epidemic proportion. It is the commonest cause of cardiovascular disability.

Risk factors for the development of CHD include a positive family history, age, genetic predisposition, abnormal blood-lipid profile, arterial hyper-tension, smoking, state of mild to severe stress and diabetes mellitus. A few other factors of importance are obesity and lack of physical activity. The patho-physiology of the disease includes plaque formation in the coronary lumen. This also happens due to excess intake of cholesterol-forming saturated fats or an abnormal lipid metabolism. These lipid-laden plaques may result in partial or complete vessel blockage, which ultimately leads to severe myocardial infarction and sudden death. To avoid the occurrence of such a critical and fatal condition, every person should educate himself/herself about the fundamental structure and functions of the heart and causative factors producing CHD.

Yoga is an ancient science whose technique is based on well-tried scientific principles. It is a science that shows how to communicate with the body, mind and soul. The trio of body, mind and soul is the basis of maintaining the state of health and well-being. Any imbalance in the functional mechanism of these faculties may result in some disease; and to reverse the state of disease to the state of health, one has to re-establish the balance in the intercommunication among the trio of body, mind and soul. This can be achieved only through yoga and meditation. Positive thinking and attiude are also essential for revival, which is also possible through yoga.

Yogic life-style and diet-style are two important aspects that play a very crucial and significant role in successfully relieving from undue pressure of deteriorating internal biochemical homeostatic conditions, which are basically responsible for several diseases including CHD. To combat and counteract the factors responsible for genesis of diseases successfully, one has to strictly and rigidly follow the yogic dietary regime, whereas by adopting basic principles of yogic life-style one can integrate one's health as well as all dimensions of one's existence, viz. physical, mental, emotional, intellectual, social and spiritual. Thus complete yogic life-style and dietary pattern will not only yield a disease-free body with sound health, but also promote the reversal of several severe diseases including CHD.

Dhyan or meditation is one of the most important components of Patanjali's integrated practice of yoga. Preksha meditation is one of the several systems of meditation. Its techniques are easy to learn, easy to perform, easy to adopt and easy to practice. Its eight components deal with basal metabolic activity of the body, functions of different body systems, vital energy, hormonal profile, concentration etc. Regular practice of all these components has shown significant effects on various physiological, biochemical and neuro-endocrinological functions of the human body. It has shown tremendous effects on mental and emotional states of the practitioner, thereby modifying the psychological state and achieving happiness, bliss and to overcome the factors of anger, ego, hatred etc.

Aiming to provide all relevant information, the book has been prepared to serve as an effective manual for the patients suffering from coronary heart disease as well as for those who want to keep CHD away. The book has been divided into six sections. Section I deals with the structure and functions of the human body and heart. In Section II patho-physiological information about CHD, factors causing CHD and its conventional management techniques have been described. Section III deals with relationship between stress and coronary heart disease, and its management. In Section IV the principles of yoga, its therapeutic basis, and its techniques related to CHD management have been elaborated. Section V contains the detailed information regarding dietary management. The last Section VI provides the details of *innovative yogic life-style intervention programme* to manage CHD. In this section procedural details of its various components are given in a systematic manner to guide the practitioner to follow the programme properly. The results of an experimental scientific study have also been included in this section as an evidence of the efficacy of the innovative yogic life-style intervention programme. Some annexures are also given in the end which provide supportive information.

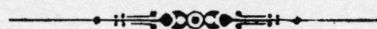

Section 1

Human Body and Heart

CHAPTER 1

Know Your Body

Contents

1.1	Human machine	9
1.2	Cell	10
1.3	Organs system	10
1.4	Skeletal system	10
1.5	Muscular system	11
1.6	Integumentary system (Skin)	11
1.7	Digestive system	11
1.8	Circulatory system	11
1.9	Respiratory system	12
1.10	Excretory system	13
1.11	Nervous system	13
1.12	Sense organs	13
1.13	Endocrine system	14
1.14	Reproductive system	14

Know Your Body

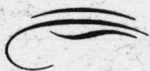

1.1 Human Machine

Strange! Everyone lives in one's own body, each moment, for the whole life, but knows very little about the structure of its vital organs, systems and their functions. Everybody should know about this machine for its proper care and maintenance as well as for its protection from various disorders and diseases.

Just as a house is built with several types of big and small bricks, cement, lime, mud etc., in the same way the body is made up of some building blocks. However, the blocks used in the body have life, whereas those used in building are lifeless. The body can also be compared to a big state. As the functions of a state can be divided into several departments and each department is independently responsible for its own functions, similarly we have various organs (departments) in our body, which perform their duties in a team spirit and perfect co-ordination. The different systems of the body and their functions are summarised here.

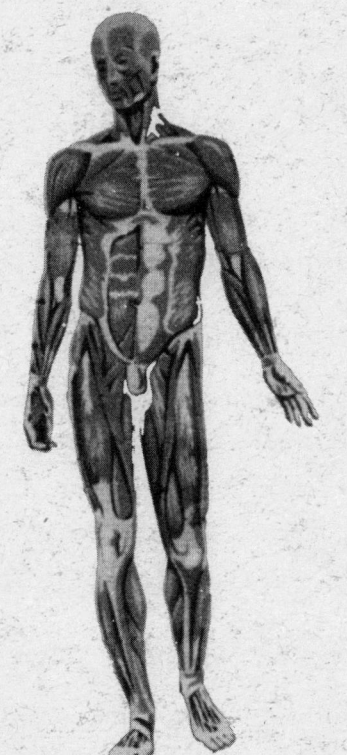

Fig. 1.1 Human Machine

The human machine is a wonderful creation and is one of the most exciting of nature's miracles.

1.2 Cell

Cells are the smallest composite units of the body, which cannot be seen with the naked eye.

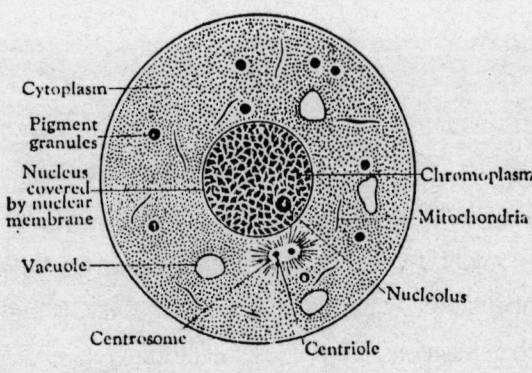

Fig. 1.2 Microscopic view of cell

The cell is often called the basic element of life. Within its confinement, thousands of chemical reactions take place. Each cell is bounded by a delicate cell membrane and at the centre of each cell is the nucleus, enclosed in its own membrane. This is the control centre without which it cannot exist. The nucleus, as its name indicates, is a very important structure. Each nucleus contains a complete set of hereditary information, encoded in the DNA blueprints. For its operation, the cell requires a lot of energy, which is generated in hundreds of super-minute power stations, called mitochondria.

This tiny fragment of life contains the `genes', the messengers of heredity. Genes are strung into long thin chains, called chromosomes. There are 46 (23 pairs) chromosomes in each human cell. DNA is the dictator of all cells, controlling their behaviour by ordering their constituents what to make, what to seek and what to avoid. It can be compared to an architect who designs, draws up plans and prepares blueprints for a building. The actual construction is carried out by the contractor, called RNA.

To sum up, the cells participate in every function of the body from birth to death. It is really a supreme wonder how 60 billion (600 kharabs) of them live in such harmony, and each one of them performs its own assigned duties.

1.3 Organ Systems

The tissues composed of cell units constitute different organs. Few organs in association with each other for similar function ultimately constitute a system. A few important systems undertaking vital body function are considered here.

1.4 Skeletal System

It provides the basic framework that supports the body. It consists of bones, cartilage and connective tissues, which bind them together. It protects the vital but vulnerable organs of the body. In an adult of average height and weight, about 206 bones work together in harmonious co-ordination with muscles and tissues, to control, support and move the limbs, which enable one to run, jump and undertake varied activities.

1.5 Muscular System

It consists of skeletal and smooth muscles. It works with the bones to provide support and to produce movements in various organs of the body. It is responsible for all the physical work being done by the body.

1.6 Integumentary System (Skin)

Skin is both a mechanical and chemical barrier between the body and the environment. It protects the body from microbes, injury to inner tissues as well as from damage by ultra-violet radiation of the sun. It also protects the body from dehydration. It retains heat in cold weather and dissipates excess heat in hot weather, and thus helps the body in temperature regulation.

1.7 Digestive System

It is concerned with the intake, break-down and absorption of food materials and the elimination of solid wastes. The important organs engaged in digestion are mouth, teeth, food pipe or oesophagus, stomach where the food is broken down and mixed with digestive juices; duodenum and small intestines (7 metres coiled) where the food constituents/nutrients are

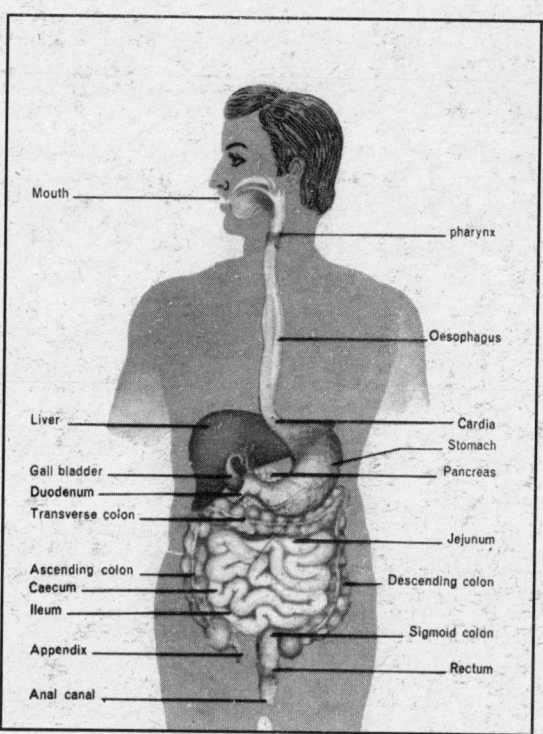

Fig. 1.3 Digestive system

absorbed in the blood stream. The large intestine is the store-house of waste material. Pancreas, liver and gall bladder are other important accessory organs of the digestive system.

1.8 Circulatory System

It distributes nutrients and oxygen to the cells and carries away their waste products. About 5 litres of blood circulates/rotates non-stop in the whole body, round the clock. Heart pumps the blood, which flows through arteries, veins and very thin capillaries to reach each and every cell of the body. The blood contains RBCs,

Yogic Cure to Avoid Heart Surgery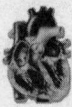

WBCs and platelets. It is purified and oxygenated in the lungs.

The oxygenated arterial blood has a bright

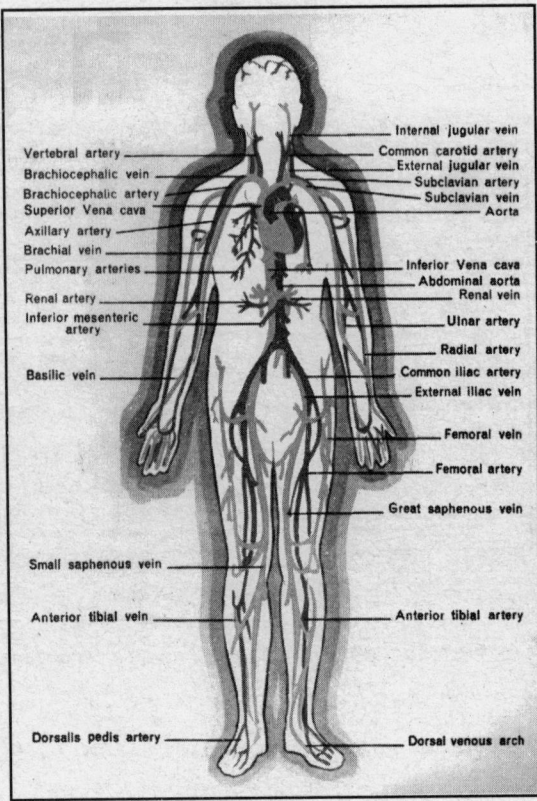

Fig. 1.4 Circulatory system

red colour, whereas that in the veins, having spent/lost its oxygen, has a bluish-purple look. Total amount of iron in RBCs is about 3 grams, but it is priceless, as one cannot live without it. White blood cells are the soldiers in the body who protect us and fight with all types of invaders till death, if need be. Platelets are the clotting cells, they are the key link in the mechanism for the prevention of blood loss.

1.9 Respiratory System

It provides the means for bringing oxygen into the body and eliminating carbon dioxide (the toxic gas). One may survive for a long time without food, for about a week without water, but one cannot last more than a few minutes without oxygen. Blood circulates and delivers the oxygen and brings the waste gases to the lungs for exchange with fresh oxygen.

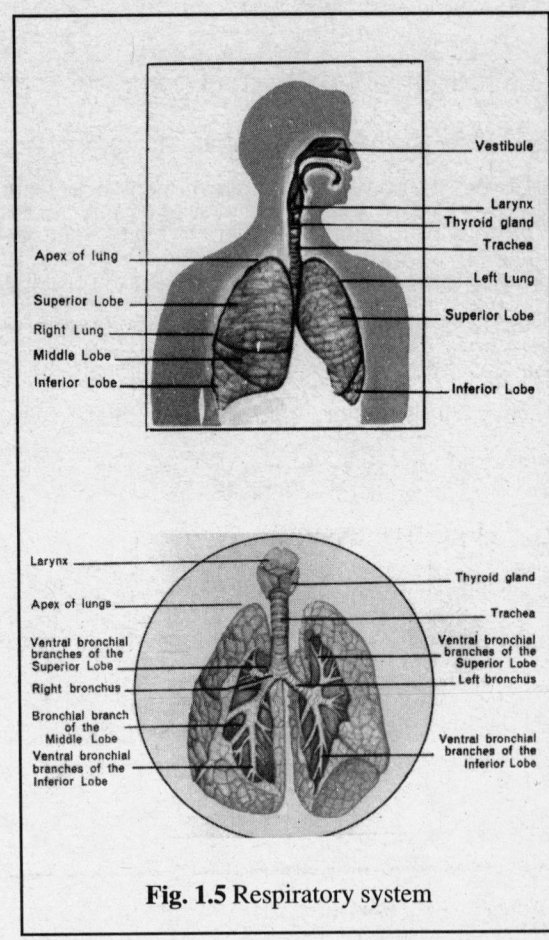

Fig. 1.5 Respiratory system

The respiratory system includes the nose, pharynx, larynx, trachea, two bronchi, bronchioles arranged in a sequence that branch and rebranch, looking like an inverted tree. The respiratory tubes end in tiny air sacs, called alveoli, in which the exchange of gases takes place. The bronchioles and alveoli constitute the lungs.

The total capacity of a lung is about 5 litres of air, but normally we breathe only 0.5 litre. Such a low amount of air reaching our lungs adversely affects upon our health due to insufficient supply of this vital life element that can be obtained simply free by adoption of proper body postures and pranayama. This can be increased by practice of complete scientific breathing, through yoga. Similarly, we take 15-16 breaths a minute, which can also be reduced by practice, by increasing the duration and quality of each breath.

1.10 Excretory System

Proper disposal of waste products is essential to keep the body clean. The excretory system works to eliminate the waste products of all the cells in the body. Lungs, skin (sweat glands), alimentary canal (large intestine) and kidneys are the main parts involved in this system.

1.11 Nervous System

The nervous system is a highly developed communication system in the human body. It co-ordinates and controls the functions of all the systems. Its failure results in total cessation of all activities, as without it one would be unable to use muscles, unable to move hands, blink eyes, to sit or stand and even to breathe. Central nervous system, peripheral nervous system and autonomous nervous system are the main divisions of the nervous system. Autonomous Nervous System (ANS) deals with the internal activities of the body, e.g. breathing, digestion, blood circulation and excretion.

The brain is the most complex and the most important part of the central nervous system. It is the site of consciousness, thought, memory, creativity, speech, vision, hearing, smell, control of endocrine glandular secretions and autonomic functions. Spinal cord is the extension (annexe) of the brain, from which originate the spinal nerves, controlling the skeletal muscles.

1.12 Sense Organs

This includes five special senses, i.e. eyes, ears, nose, mouth and the entire skin surface, with receptors for collecting and conveying useful information from the environment to the brain. Human senses include hearing, sight, smell, taste and touch. The eyes function as a mechanical camera, sending information about visual objects and are capable of detecting light, shades of colours, degrees of light and darkness, besides being extremely expressive of moods and emotions. The ears are two organs in one. They are organs of hearing and perception of sound as well as centres of co-ordination. The function of sense of smell is performed by the nose in attraction of food and warning of danger. Taste buds found on the tongue respond to chemical substances dissolved in saliva on the surface of the tongue. It is performed inside the mouth. Touch sensation results from stimulation of tactile nerves, which convey infromation regarding the size and shape of the object, hot or cold or any substance favourable or unfavourable to our body.

The controller of all sense organs is the brain, which senses them through a variety of receptors. Sense organs have no significance until the sensory waves reach the brain. Thus we actually perceive all sensations in the brain. In short, it is not the eye that see, but the brain, which sees through the eye organ. Same is the case with other senses.

1.13 Endocrine System

It comprises a few specialised endocrine glands, which produce chemical substances (hormones) that affect other cells and organs and help control and co-ordinate their activities. Main glands are Pineal, Pituitary, Thyroid, Parathyroid, Thymus, Adrenal, Gonads and Pancreas. Pancreas produces insulin to convert glucose into glycogen and it keeps the body's sugar at a normal level. There are other hormones too, secreted by these glands, which form the nature and habits of a person.

1.14 Reproductive System

This system functions for the continuation of species. The males produce sperm and the females produce ovum. When fertilization occurs, both these cells combine and as a result new cell is formed that is genetically complete. This new cell later on gradually develops into a complete human being.

CHAPTER 2

Know Your Heart

Contents

2.1	Introduction	17
2.2	Structure of heart	17
2.3	Heart : miracle pump	17
2.4	Blood circulation	18
2.5	Four heart chambers	19
2.6	Four major heart valves	20
2.7	Blood vessels — arteries, capillaries	21
2.8	Pulmonary veins and arteries	21
2.9	Aorta	22
2.10	Nourishment of heart and coronary arteries	22
2.11	Cardiac output	22
2.12	Blood stream and composition of blood	23
2.13	Heart beat and pulse	23

Know Your Heart

2.1 Introduction

The heart is a very efficient instrument (organ) that performs a great role in human life. If the heart stops to work or all hearts of the world form a union and go on strike even for a few minutes or so, the whole functioning of the body will come to a standstill and not a single living being will remain alive, and this whole earth would be converted into a heap of dead bodies all around. Most of the hearts work, as they are expected to, but why do some hearts react differently? What makes them indifferent to the body's needs or behave abnormally than others? Who is to blame? The heart itself, its genes, environment where the person lives, his/her style of living, the modern system of health maintenance, the food and medicines the person takes, improper nourishment or the improper education? These are some of the basic questions that need some heart searching.

2.2 Structure of Heart

The human heart is a small muscular organ situated in the centre of the chest, a little to the left side. In size, it is roughly that of a clenched fist and in weight it is about 350 grams. As it is such an important and delicate part of the body, it is protected by the sternum (breast bone) in front. The heart retains its priority among all important organs of the human body by the fact that it is responsible for supplying blood, oxygen and other nutrients to the entire system of human machinery.

Its function is like a pump that never stops nor tires while performing its duty day and night without any rest or break during the whole life period of about 70-75 years.

2.3 Heart : a Miracle Pump

If a salesman shows you a miracle pump, which can pump about 700 million litres of liquid to keep your factory running, you may not

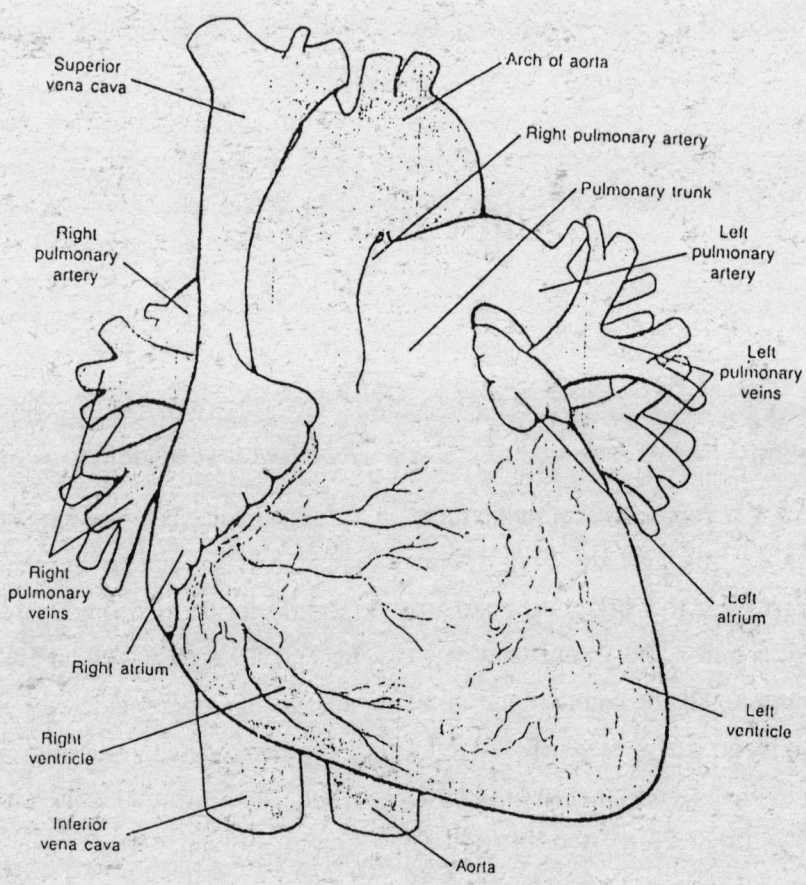

Fig. 2.1 Heart : external structure

believe it. But the human heart is just a miracle pump that circulates the blood, 1 lakh kilometres every day.

Internally the heart is divided into four chambers. The right two chambers contain impure blood and the left two contain pure one. These are separated by a septum (a wall between the right and left chambers) which does not allow the blood on either side to get mixed. Further, the heart is equipped with 4 major valves, which function to allow the blood to flow in one direction only.

2.4 Blood Circulation

Blood is the essence of life. It is always circulating non-stop in the body and is responsible for transporting energy, hormones, chemicals, nutrients and raw materials to each and every cell/tissue in the body and clears away the waste products to keep body cells alive. This transporting system is called blood circulation system. The heart is responsible for the drive/push. With every contraction, expansion or beat of the heart a specific volume of blood is driven into the blood stream through the arteries (big vessels), arterioles (smaller vessels), capillaries (thin vessels), tissues and cells.

When the muscular tissue of the heart contracts, the chamber concerned becomes smaller and, as a result, the presure in the cavities grows and the blood is pushed into the direction where the pressure is lower. The heart valves ensure absolute one-way traffic. When the left ventricle of the heart pushes the blood under high pressure, the blood flows through the arteries of circulatory system to the capillary network of the body to supply oxygen and other nutrients to the tissues/cells and to remove the waste products therefrom.

The blood carrying the wastes returns again to the heart via the veins and enters the right atrium and then the right ventricle. It takes the reverse route: cells, tissues, capillaries, veinlets, veins. The blood is then pumped into the capillary network of the lungs through the arteries of pulmonary circuit. This blood after it is duly purified in the lungs, returns to the heart via the pulmonary veins and enters the left atrium. The left atrium then pushes the blood into the left ventricle. The circle is thus completed. It may be noted that both the atria (right and left) are active at the same time and later both the ventricles are active at the same time.

As pointed out earlier, the heart is actually a dual action pump, once to send the blood into the lungs and then to push it into the body. The first is a short loop connection from the heart to the lungs and back after purification, and the second a long loop branching from the heart to supply blood to all parts of the body and uniting again to reach ultimatly the heart. Both the circuits start and end in the heart and there is no mixing of blood between them.

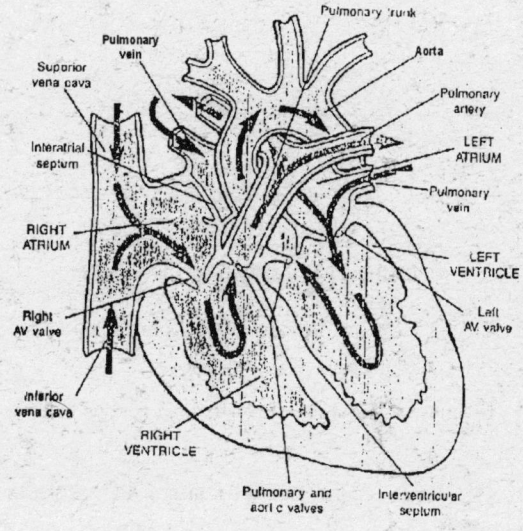

Fig.2.2 Heart : Diagrammatic section. Arrows show the direction of blood flow.

2.5 Four Heart Chambers

There are four chambers in the heart, two at right side and two at left. The upper chambers are called 'atria' and the lower ones are called 'ventricles'. Right atrium and ventricle deal with impure blood whereas left atrium and ventricle deal with oxygenated and pure blood.

Yogic Cure to Avoid Heart Surgery

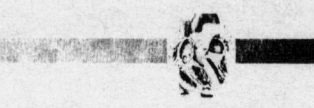

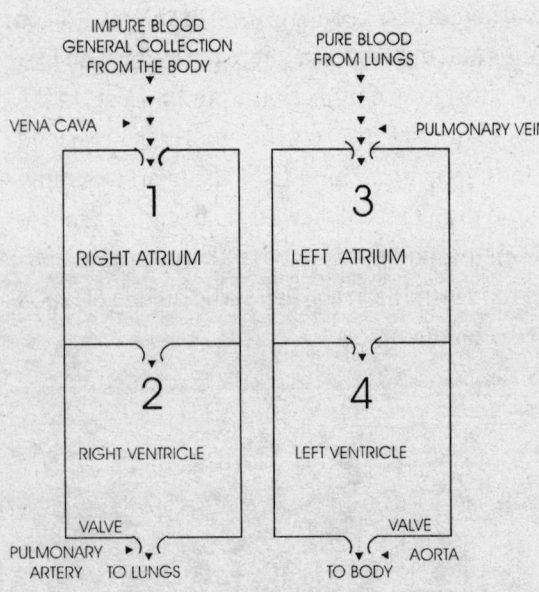

Fig. 2.3 Schematic representation of heart chambers. Arrows indicate direction of blood flow

1. **Tricuspid valve :** Located between the right atrium and right ventricle, allows blood to flow towards the right ventricle.

2. **Mitral valve :** Located between the left atrium and left ventricle; allows blood flow towards left ventricle.

3. **Pulmonary valve :** Located between the right ventricle and pulmonary artery, which allows blood to flow towards pulmonary region.

4. **Aortic valve :** Located between the left ventricle and aorta; allows blood to flow towards the aorta and body.

(These valves allow blood to flow in one direction only. The blood cannot return through these valves).

Chamber 1: Gets impure blood from the body and pushes it to chamber no. 2.

Chamber 2 : Sends the blood to lungs for purification and oxygenation.

Chamber 3 : Gets purified blood from the lungs and pushes it into chamber no. 4.

Chamber 4 : Strongest and most useful chamber. It pushes the pure blood again into the whole body including the heart, through the aorta.

2.6 Four Major Heart Valves

There are 4 major valves functioning in the heart. The valves fitted between atria and ventricles are called the atrio-ventricular (AV) valves and those between ventricles and major arteries (aorta and pulmonary artery) are called arterial valves.

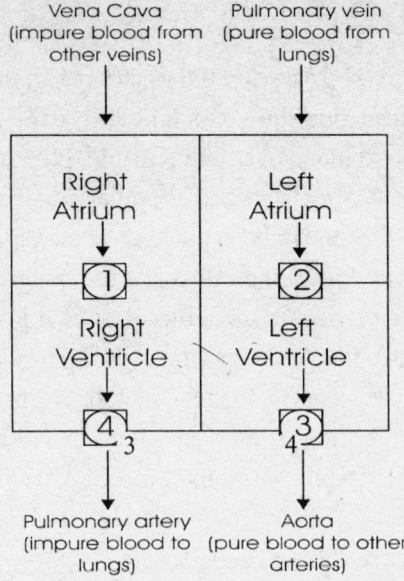

Fig. 2.4 Diagram of heart valve chambers

Blood Circulation inside the Heart

The blood circulation is one way only and the heart is always working non-stop, even during the sleep.

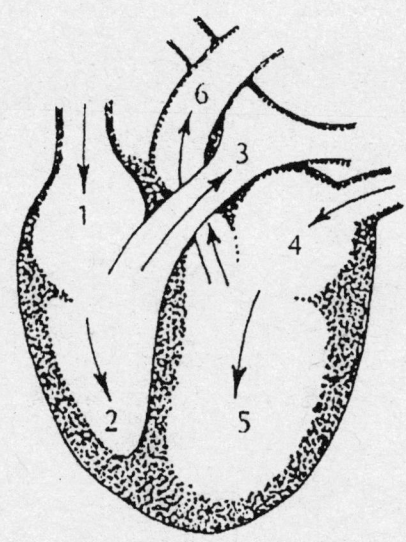

Fig. 2.5 Circulation of blood inside heart

1. Impure blood enters the right atrium from vena cava.
2. From the right atrium (1), impure blood goes into the right ventricle (2).
3. Impure blood reaches the lungs through the pulmonary artery.
4. Pure blood comes to the left atrium from the lungs through the pulmonary vein.
5. From the left atrium, pure blood enters the left ventricle (5).
6. Aorta takes pure blood to the whole body

2.7 Blood Vessels— Arteries, Veins, Capillaries

The vessels through which the blood travels are called arteries, veins and capillaries. There are more than 1 lakh kilometres long blood vessels functioning in the human body. Their interconnected network reaches practically each and every cell of the body. The blood vessels carrying the blood from the heart to the body are called arteries, whereas those carrying the blood in the opposite direction, i.e. towards the heart, are named veins.

Oxygenated blood leaves the heart chambers via aorta, which emerges from the left ventricle and soon branches into two—one going upwards to the heart and the second downwards to the trunk and limbs. Aorta is divided into arteries (big vessels) and again into arterioles (smaller vessels) and then into thin-walled capillaries. Capillaries are so small (0.006 mm dia- meter) that red blood corpuscles (RBCs) have to pass through them one by one in a single profile.

Oxygen, food materials and hormones transported in the blood are transferred into cells, whereas all waste products are diffused into the blood to be excreted outside the body. The exchange is so rapid that each blood unit spends only a couple of seconds or so in a particular capillary.

2.8 Pulmonary Veins and Arteries

Both these blood vessels are the main routes to join the heart and lungs. The pulmonary artery takes the impure blood from the heart and sends it to the lungs, where it is purified. The pulmonary vein brings pure blood from the lungs to the heart.

Vena cava is the largest vein, which receives the impure blood from the body and pushes it into the right atrium. It works in two ways, one to receive impure blood from the upper part and the second to bring impure blood from the lower portion of the body.

2.9 Aorta

Aorta is the largest artery in the body. Blood from the left ventricle is pushed into the aorta, from where it travels into other arteries, arterioles and capillaries in the whole body. The arteries supplying the nourishment to the heart are called coronary arteries. They also originate from the aorta.

2.10 Nourishment of Heart and Coronary Arteries

As already explained, the heart is continuously working and has to perform the great role of transporting blood to each and every cell of the body to keep the person alive. It also requires proper nourishment, i.e. blood, oxygen, glucose etc. Though the heart deals with thousands of litres of blood daily, it cannot use single drop of the blood passing through its chambers for its own use. The heart, like a honest cashier, has to depend for its nourishment upon its own share and the special arteries responsible to feed the heart are the coronary arteries.

There are two coronary arteries (left and right), which originate from the aorta. The left further branches into two just after its origin, (i) left anterior descending artery and (ii) left circumflex coronary artery. All these coronary arteries are connected with each other and are distributed into many smaller vessels all over the heart surface. The blockage or narrowing in these arteries is the main cause of hypertension (high blood pressure), angina, CHD and heart attack.

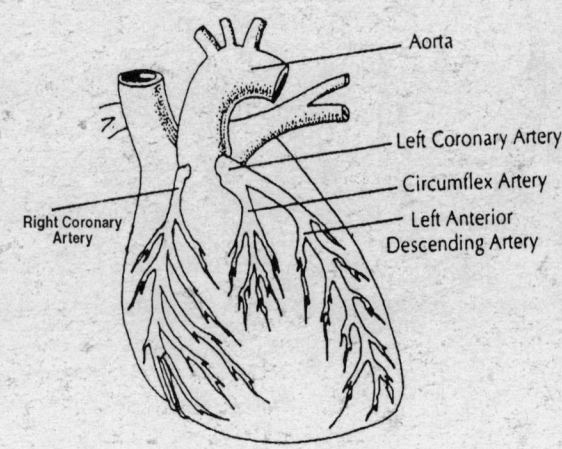

Fig. 2.6 Coronary arteries

2.11 Cardiac Output

With an average heart beat of 70-72 per minute, the cardiac output comes to about 5 litres of blood. Thus in the span of just 1 minute, a volume equivalent to all the blood in the body passes through the heart. During excessive physical work or mental stress, this function increases five-folds or even more.

An average adult has 4.5 to 5 litres blood

circulating in the system. It has been estimated that during a man's life time about 50 crore litres of blood is pumped or transported. Normally the liver receives 28%, the kidneys 24% and muscles 15% blood. It is consumed by brain 14%, the heart 5% and the remaining is consumed by other parts of the body.

2.12 Blood Stream and Composition of Blood

Blood is the carrier-vehicle through which, besides oxygen, a variety of other substances like glucose, fats, amino acids, water, salts, minerals, vitamins, hormones etc. are delivered to all the cells and tissues to keep them alive and vigorous. At the same time, carbon dioxide and other waste materials are also carried to the lungs, kidneys etc. for their excretion.

Blood is composed of about 55% fluid and 45% solid matter. One drop of blood contains about 250 million blood cells. The main components of blood are red blood cells (RBC), white blood cells (WBC) and platelets (clotting cells).

There are 5 million RBCs in 1 mm^3 blood. A red cell has an average life-span of 120 days, during which it makes 3 lakh trips, travelling more than a 1,000 km. Haemoglobin is its important constituent, containing iron. It has a strong affinity for oxygen. When red cells come into contact with oxygen, they take it up to form oxy-haemoglobin. The oxygenated blood (blood mixed with oxygen) has a bright red colour. When it reaches the cells, the oxygen reacts with carbon to form carboxy-haemoglobin, which is bluish purple in colour. This again, on reaching the lungs, gets a fresh supply of oxygen and liberates carbon dioxide. The cycle thus continues. The haemoglobin content of blood provides an index of an individual's health.

White blood cells (WBC) are our body-guards. These are colourless and do not contain haemoglobin, but they are larger than RBCs and move more actively. In fact they are the fighting soldiers and perfom their duties outside the actual blood in the neighbourhood of tissues. They are our military force that fight against foreign invaders like bacteria and viruses. Then there are platelets, which help prevent the loss of blood through clotting.

All these constituents are mixed in the liquid portion of the blood, called plasma. This blood circulates throughout the body in long, narrow blood vessels (arteries and veins), being regulated by the master switch, the heart.

2.13 Heart Beat and Pulse

As and when the heart pumps the blood and pushes it, a wave of pressure travels along the walls of arteries, which can be observed or felt as pulse. With every expansion and contraction

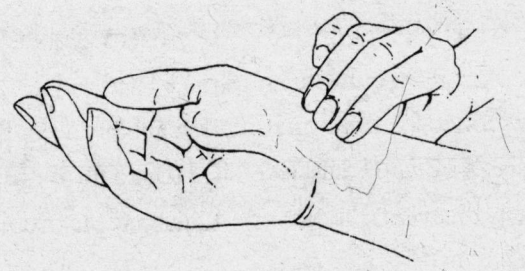

Fig. 2.7 Radial artery in the wrist

of the heart, a throbbing or vibration is produced in the arteries, which is called 'heart beat' or 'pulse'. The pulse can be felt at places on the surface of the body where the artery is more superficial or nearer to the surface. Normally the pulse is felt on the inner surface of the wrist below the thumb.

Normal pulse rate

New born	:	130-140 per minute
3 years	:	95-100 per minute
8 years	:	80-95 per minute
Adults	:	72 per minute
Aged persons	:	72-76 per minute

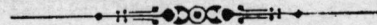

CHAPTER 3

Cardiac Problems

Contents

3.1	Angina	27
3.2	Heart attack	27
3.3	How to recognise angina and heart attack	28
3.4	Hypertension (high blood pressure)	28
3.5	Systolic and diastolic pressure	28
3.6	Prevention of heart attack, angina and hypertension	28

➢ Yogic life-style, diet control, regular physical exercise, avoid mental tension, stop smoking, regular medical check-up

Cardiac Problems

3.1 Angina

Angina pain refers to the chest pain caused by inadequate blood supply to the heart. The term 'angina' comes from a Greek word, meaning 'to choke'. Angina is regarded as a symptom of coronary artery disease. For proper functioning of the heart, the heart muscles also need oxygen and essential nutrients. When the arteries due to fat or cholesterol deposits become narrow, the obstruction (called athero-sclerosis) leads to insufficient blood supply to the heart. Consequently angina occurs. The process of atherosclerosis however starts in early childhood and gradually progresses.

Anginal attacks are often caused due to excessive physical exertion or emotional upsets such as climbing stairs after meals, walking up the hill, heavy meals, smoking, anger, excitement, fear or similar negative emotions etc. The chest pain of angina is recurrent and short lived (5 to 10 minutes).

3.2 Heart Attack

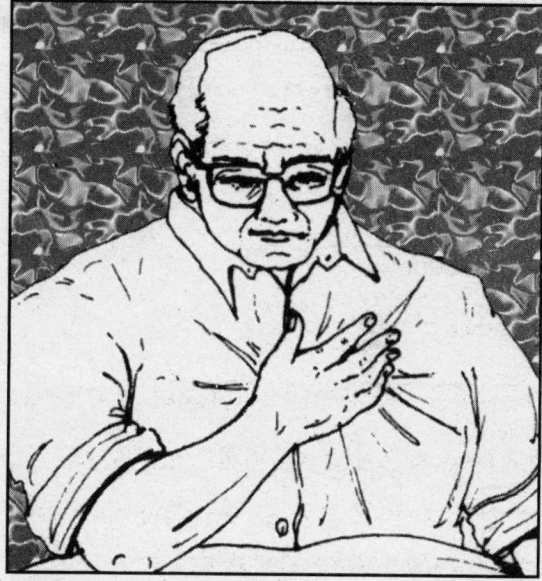

Fig. 3.1 A person under the state of heart attack

When any of the coronary arteries gets completely blocked, the specific part of heart (heart muscle tissue) being fed by that artery does not receive oxygen and it dies. This is called **myocardial infarction,** and consequently a heart attack occurs that may prove fatal. A tablet of 'sorbitrate' is used for its immediate cure.

3.3 How to Recognise Angina and Heart Attack

The major symptoms of angina are the following:

1. Chest pain, mild or severe : It usually occurs in the centre of the chest and radiates to the left arm, though occasionally to the right arm also and even to the lower jaw.
2. Nausea (sense of vomiting) or actual vomiting.
3. Pain or unusual heaviness in upper abdomen with sensation of fullness (gas) in chest.
4. Breathlessness or short breath.
5. Sweating.
6. Weakness.
7. Fainting and dizziness.
8. Choking sensation in the throat.

3.4 Hypertension (High Blood Pressure)

Blood pressure is the pressure put on the walls of the arteries, due to the flow of blood through them, on being pumped by the heart. Blood pressure varies from time to time. It may rise at the time of excitement and may decrease when one is calm and at rest. Hypertension is a very common disease, affecting about 25 per cent of adults all over the world. As a majority of the people are unaware of it or do not attach proper importance to it, it is called a silent killer.

Continued high blood pressure forces the heart and circulatory system to overwork. As a result, the heart becomes enlarged, leading to its failure besides stroke (brain haemorrhage), damage to kidney or eyes, and other psychosomatic diseases like diabetes, ulcers etc.

3.5 Systolic and Diastolic Pressure

Blood pressure is the measurement of the pressure exerted by blood on blood vessels (arteries). It is measured in terms of mm of Hg (mercury).

Blood pressure is of two types, i.e. (i) systolic and (ii) diastolic. Systolic pressure is the pressure exerted by the blood during contraction of the heart, while diastolic pressure is the pressure exerted by blood when the heart is relaxing (heart is at rest). As diastolic is the one which is present all the time, it is of more importance than systolic pressure. B.P. varies because of many reasons, the most important being age and sex.

Average normal or desirable blood pressure:

For young people : 120/80

For old people : 140/90

3.6 Prevention of Heart Attack, Angina and Hypertension

Prevention refers to our style of life. The prevention must start in early childhood, because atherosclerosis (deposition of fat or cholesterol in coronary arteries) also starts at the same time.

The following are some steps to be taken to avoid CHD.

(1) **Yogic life style** : Yogic life style interventions include relaxation, diet modification, avoiding worry, stress or mental tension, regular exercise and walking, some meditation or to remember God and to live a disciplined and cheerful life.

(2) **Diet control :** Food containing cholesterol should be avoided like eggs, ghee, butter and cream products. Instead one should use mustard oil, corn oil, or soybean oil. High fibrous vegetarian diet, vegetables and fruits reduce heart attacks and angina. To avoid overweight one should never overeat or take excessive coffee, tea or alcohol.

To prevent hypertension and diabetes, too much salt and sugar should be avoided. Balanced vegetarian diet is good and healthy.

(3) **Regular physical exercise :** One should perform physical yogic exercises everyday. Walking, jogging etc. are also equally good. Regular exercise, asanas and pranayama also prevent obesity and joint diseases, besides keeping the blood cholesterol at normal levels.

(4) **Avoid mental tension :** Mental tension and stress add to athero-sclerosis (artery blockage). One should avoid a sedentary life, check emotional stress and try to live a tension free, peaceful life.

(5) **Stop smoking :** Smoking increases roughness in the walls of arteries and formation of coronary thrombosis (blockage) besides lung diseases and ulcers. Even smoking of cigarette is harmful to the heart. Smoking of cigars, bidis and chewing tobacco are equally harmful.

(6) **Regular medical check-up :** To prevent heart attack, periodical medical check-up is necessary in respect of B.P., ECG, blood sugar and cholesterol level. Any abnormality detected should be peroperly attended to.

Six golden rules for prevention :

1. Yogic life style.
2. Proper diet.
3. Regular exercise.
4. Avoiding stress or tension.
5. No smoking.
6. Periodical medical chek-up.

Section 2

Coronary Heart Disease

CHAPTER 4

Coronary Heart Disease

Contents

4.1	Introduction	35
4.2	Coronary thrombosis	35
4.3	Conventional management of CHD	36
4.4	Medical management	36
	➢ Vasodilators, anti-platelet drugs, drugs that reduce oxygen demand of heart	
4.5	Surgical management	37
	➢ Pace-maker, angioplasty, bypass surgery (open-heart surgery)	

Coronary Heart Disease

4.1 Introduction

The coronary heart disease (CHD), also called coronary artery disease (CAD) or ischaemic heart disease (IHD) is one of the leading causes of mortality and morbidity throughout the world. Now it is on a constant rise in our country too. The main cause of this disease is deposition of cholesterol and fat on the inner smooth lining of the blood vessels (coronary arteries), resulting in their blockage and obstruction in the flow of blood through them. An atheromatous plaque is formed, which restricts the flow of blood, oxygen and nutrients to the heart.

When blockage in the coronary arteries reaches more than 60 to 70 per cent, under exertion the increased demand of blood supply by the heart is not met with, and a sensation of pain is felt in the chest, which may also move down the left arm, typically called angina. This is a very dreadful condition, and if left unattended it may threaten life. However a 70% or more blockage does not develop in a day or a couple of months or years, it takes about 30 to 40 years to reach a stage when it can be detected.

4.2 Coronary Thrombosis

Blockage in the coronary artery due to fomation of blood clots is called `coronary thrombosis'. When blood clots are formed in the arteries by sticking of platelets, red blood cells and other cells together, the walls of the arteries become weak, brittle and roughened, causing an obstruction in the blood flow. A particular coronary artery becomes narrow and the heart does not get the proper nourishment. Consequently hypertension, angina and heart attack occur.

Thrombosis occurs not only in coronary arteries but also in any other artery of the body. If the blood clot is formed in the artery going toward the brain, brain haemorrhage follows. This is termed `stroke', which may lead to paralysis and even instant death. Smokers suffer from thrombosis more than non-smokers. Thrombosis

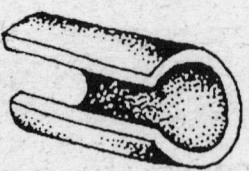

(A)
Fig.4.1 Healthy artery : In early childhood, the artery walls are free of any damage

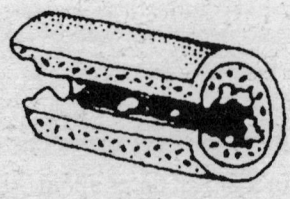

(B)
Fig.4.1 Atherosclerosis : In later years arteries become clogged with plaque due to factors such as excessive cholesterol

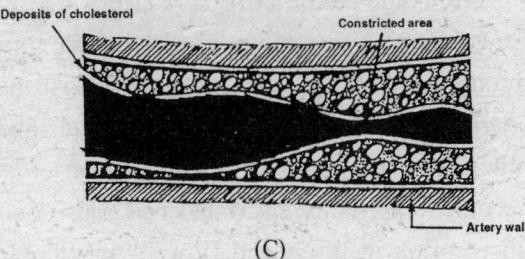

(C)
Fig.4.1 Longitudnal cross-section of an artery showing variation of cholesterol deposition along the artery wall

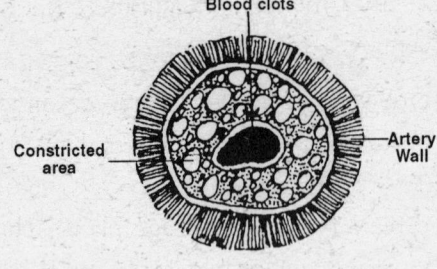

(D)
Fig.4.1 Blood clot formation in the constricted area of artery

can be prevented to some extent by lessening the over-load of work, physical exertion, avoiding excitement and stress, reducing a cholesterol-ful diet and by leading a yogic and more regulated life.

4.3 Conventional Management of CHD

Conventional management of CHD comprises two important techniques :

(i) Medical Management

(ii) Surgical Management.

4.4 Medical Management

Till date coronary heart diseases are being treated with drugs (medicines), which result only in a temporary relief of symptoms. They, in no circumstances, bring about a permanent cure, as the cholesterol blockages in the coronary blood vessels are left unaffected. As a matter of fact, these blockages continue to keep on increasing in size till the rate of cholesterol deposition is reduced. Most of the drugs employed in the treatment of coronary artery disease bring about temporary relief of symptoms through one of the following actions :

(1) **Vasodilators :** Some medicines dilate the coronary blood vessels, thus increasing their luminal size and bringing about an increase of blood flow through them. These drugs have a duration of action amounting to only a few hours, and when their effect has

finished the coronary blood vessels once again attain their normal size by shrinking. In order to maintain the dilation, another doze has to be taken. The process goes on increasing with the simultaneous increase in blockages.

(2) **Anti-platelet drugs :** These drugs reduce the viscosity of blood. In other words they make the blood thin, which then is able to easily pass through the narrow space between the blockages.

(3) **Drugs that reduce oxygen demand of heart** : This is another group of medicines that decreases the oxygen demand of the heart, thus enabling the heart to do more work in the compromised amount of blood it recieves due to the blockages.

Nearly all the drugs used by cardiologists to treat coronary heart disease are being selected from one of the above groups, and from our understanding about their mode of action it is clear that all of them bring about a temporary relief from CHD symptoms, leaving the blockage as it is. In fact, they add considerably to the disease by their side effects. During the mean time, the disease process goes on increasing gradully. Our medication is also consequently increased, with no cure. Soon after, the rosy picture fades away, and once again we find ourselves back to where we had started from, and we realize that every effort we had gone through was all in vain.

As has been said, 'Dard badhta gaya, jyon jyon dava ki', that is 'pain kept on increasing as with the increase in doze and quantity of medicines'.

4.5 Surgical Management

Over the past few decades surgery has held a key position in the management of coronary heart disease. These surgical interventions are in the form of **coronary bypass surgery and angioplasty.** In spite of being an extremely abusive and expensive procedure, the results of this treatment still remain only temporary. The blocks reoccur within 2 to 3 years of angioplasty and 2 to 5 years of bypass surgery, resulting once again in the same problem in spite of much trauma and expense that has gone waste. Surgical interventions have to be complemented by invasive imaging techniques such as angiography, which is required to determine the location and extent of blockage within the coronary arteries. Angiography in itself has a long list of complications and risks, which pose a great threat to life.

Pace-maker : Pace-maker is a device fitted inside or outside the chest of the patient to regulate the irregular heart beat. It is usually equipped with a battery, which lasts for several years.

Angioplasty : Angioplasty is a technique of surgery, where a catheter tube, fitted with a balloon on its mouth, is inserted in the coronary artery of the heart where the blockage has been formed. The blockage is cleaned by inflating the balloon. This is also termed 'ballooning'.

The catheter used in angioplasty is a plastic or rubber tube, which is very fine, long and flexible. It is inserted into an artery in the arm or groin (thigh's upper joint) and pushed very gently to reach the heart. Now a days a stent is put and fixed through which the blood may flow easily.

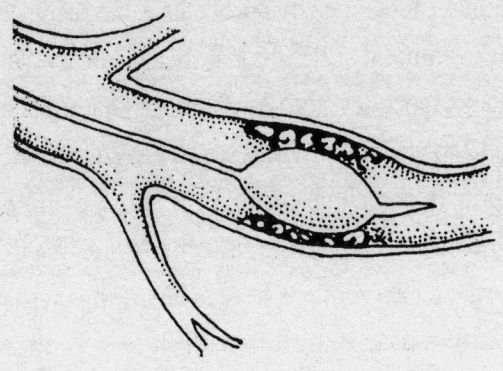

Fig. 4.2 Ballooning

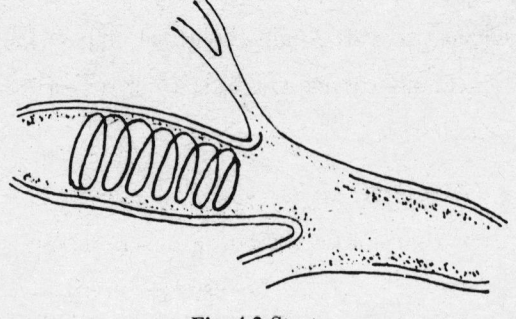

Fig. 4.3 Stent

Bypass surgery (open-heart surgery) :
Bypass surgery is a surgical technique where the blocked coronary artery is replaced with a new one by fixing it parallel to the previous defective artery. After it is fitted, the blocked portion of the original artery is left idle as it is, and the blood traffic feeding the heart is diverted through the newly stitched, successor artery.

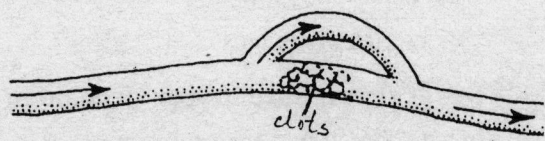

Fig. 4.4 Bypass surgery

The substitute artery used for grafting is taken from the patient's own body, as the human body does not accept the arteries or veins of another person. The successor artery for bypass is removed from the saphenous vein (from leg), radial artery (near the wrist), or mammary artery (from behind the breast bone). One end of the removed substitute artery or vein is attached to the aorta and the other end is connected below the blockage, bypassing the obstructed area.

During surgery, the blocked segment of the artery is bypassed, and thus the patient is relieved from angina/heart attack. The blockage however may reoccur, if one does not follow or observe

Coronary Heart Disease

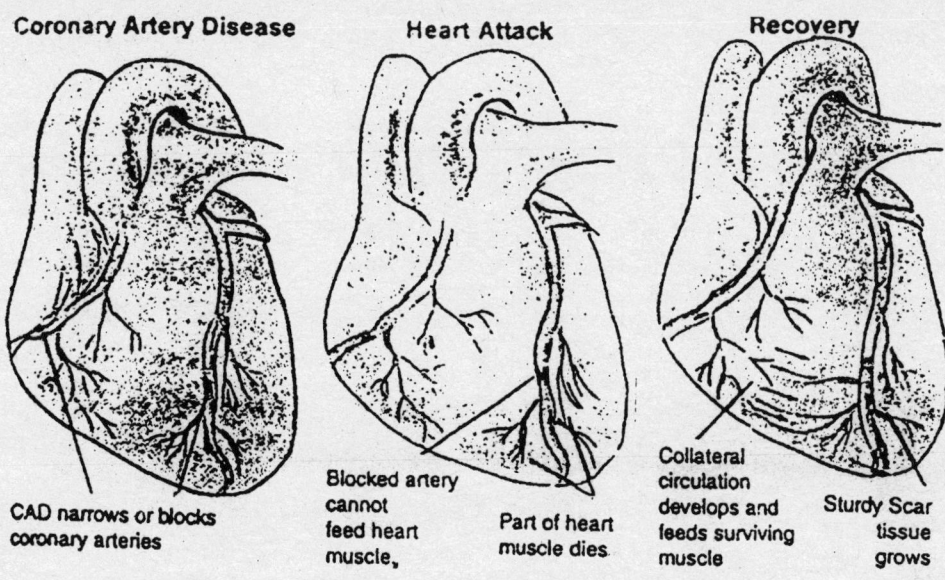

Fig. 4.5 Coronary artery disease : process and recovery

the desired precautions. Instead of changing the arteries through bypass, we should change our life style to avoid the unpleasant situation of this surgery.

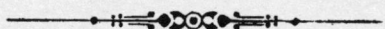

CHAPTER 5

Diagnostic Techniques for Coronary Heart Disease

Contents

5.1	Common diagnostic devices	43
5.2	ECG (Electrocardiogram)	43
5.3	Blood test (lipid profile test)	43
5.4	Echocardiography (Ultrasound Scan)	44
5.5	T.M.T. (Stress test)	44
5.6	Thallium scan	45
5.7	Pet scan	45
5.8	Angiography	45
5.9	Possible drawbacks and complications of angiography	45
5.10	Commercialisation of angiography	46
5.11	Other chest pains and angina	46

> Muscular chest pain, cervical pain in left or right arm, gastric pain in chest

Diagnostic Techniques for Coronary Heart Disease

5.1 Common Diagnostic Devices

Normally when the doctor suspects/ indicates about the heart disease, the patient feels shocked and panicky. He is confused about what to do and what not to do. Some are perturbed whereas others do not take the situation seriously and ignore it. However, both the actions are improper. The other diseases, e.g. muscular chest pain, cervical pain and gastric chest pain, sometimes due to resembalance of symptoms, are confused with angina pain. The tests mentioned below may be undertaken for correct diagnosis and to assess the severity of the disease.

5.2. ECG (Electrocardiogram)

ECG (Electrocardiogram) is an electrical recording of the heart's functioning. It reflects the deficiency of oxygen supply to the heart muscles, their blood supply, heart size, valve defects and increased heart rate. However, it gives no information about coronary blockage. It is the simplest test among all the tests to detect angina. But the analysis of ECG recording is quite difficult and is a specialized job, requiring an expert doctor for the purpose.

After listening to the brief history and checking the B.P. and pulse rate of the patient, the doctor immediately advises an ECG to ascertain the emergency. If there is no emergency, the next step should be to go for the blood tests for conducting further tests and continuing the treatment (i.e. Echo and TMT).

5.3 Blood Test (Lipid Profile Test)

As already explained in the previous chapter, the main cause of heart disease is the deposition of fat (cholesterol) in the coronary arteries. Fat exists in different forms, running in the blood stream (blood vessels). Fat components are cholesterol, triglycerides, HDL (high-density lipoprotein, a good cholesterol), and the LDL (low-density lipoprotein) and VLDL (very low-density lipoprotein, the bad cholesterols).

Therefore the blood test is essential to continue the treatment of heart disease further.

The diabetic patients are further required to get their blood glucose tested, i.e. fasting and PP. The blood sample for fasting should be collected after 12 hours of fasting, and in case of PP after 2 hours of breakfast.

Normal range of blood components per mg/dl :

Blood cholesterol	125 to 200
Triglycerides	60 to 150
LDL (bad cholesterol)	50 to 125
VLDL (very bad cholesterol)	10 to 35
HDL (good cholesterol)	30 to 60
Blood sugar/glucose (F)	75 to 110
Blood sugar/glucose (PP)	125 to 150

5.4 Echocardiography (Ultrasound Scan)

An echocardiogram also known as 'Echo test' helps the doctor to determine the structure and functions of all parts of the heart. The machine has a microphone-like device called 'Transducer'. The transducer is placed on the chest wall of the patient and it gives out ultrasound waves. The machine converts the echo sound into a graph.

This non-invasive test measures the size, shape and functioning condition of the heart and its valves besides determining the extent of functional loss or damage of the heart on account of a previous heart attack or disease. This test is also widely available.

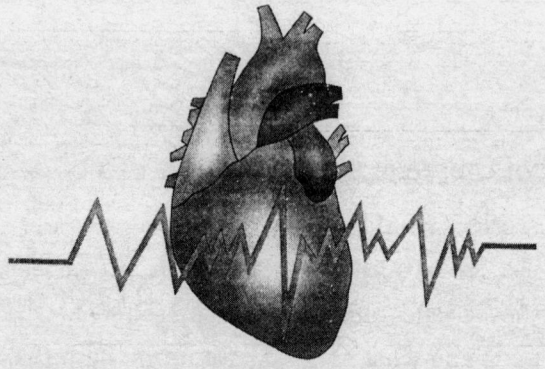

Fig.5.1 Recording of electrical currents of heart

5.5 T.M.T. (Stress Test)

Tread mill test measures the supply of oxygen to the heart. The patient has to physically exert in this test under controlled condions and a computerised machine is used to measure the rate of oxygen supply to the heart. The level of exercise is gradually increased while taking the ECG continuously, which reflects any oxygen deficit in heart muscles. Exercise is stopped as soon as the ECG shows any change or the patient feels any chest pain or breathing discomfort. If the ECG reflects early changes during exercise, the CHD is severe, and if late the disease is treated to be mild. A TMT costs around Rs 1,500 and is widely available.

5.6 Thallium Scan

The thallium scan of the heart is a little more advanced test than TMT. This test is also processed on TMT pattern but the patient is injected with a radio-labelled chemical and placed under a nuclear camera to get internal photographs. This test assesses the blood flow to heart muscles during exercise or at rest and detects the severity of CHD more accurately than TMT. This test is, however, available in selected hospitals.

5.7 Pet Scan

Pet scan is the latest investigation device to ascertain the coronary artery blockages. The patient is made to lie down on a table, which is introduced into the scanner and sectional pictures of the heart are taken to have an accurate idea of the blockages present.

5.8 Angiography

Angiography is an invasive test undertaken to assess the shape, size, exact location and gravity of the blockage in the coronary arteries. The test helps decide the position regarding surgery to bypass the diseased and obstructed portion. After injecting anaesthesia intravenously, a long tube called 'catheter' is inserted and pushed into an artery in the thigh of the patient till it reaches the heart and coronary arteries. A radio-active dye is injected through the hole in the catheter inside the coronary arteries and a series of X-rays are taken, which can be seen on the monitor. The lack of filling the coronary artery reveals the exact extent of blockage(s), which is expressed in percentage.

If the dye fills the coronary tube fully, the chances of blockage are nil, and if the dye does not fill the tube or fills a part thereof, the blockage is taken to be present. A rough percentage of blockage is then decided, i.e. 60%, 70%, 80% or more. usually it is 70% to 90%. Normally a blockage under 70% does not reflect any symptoms of CHD and the person appears quite normal.

Angiography is available in most of the centres throughout the country, and costs around Rs 15,000.

5.9 Possible Drawbacks and Complications of Angiography

1. Invasive procedure.
2. High cost.
3. Injuries possible due to damages inside the arteries while inserting and pushing the catheter.
4. Perforation in arteries, encouraging blockages.
5. Possibility of coronary artery damage.
6. Causes psychological stress.
7. Chances of re-blockage.

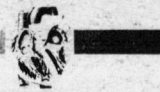

5.10 Commercialization of Angiography

Now-a-days some cardiologists have taken the angiography as a tool of spreading panic in the patient and among his/her kith and kins. They try to make the patient ready to get operated for bypass surgery, in order to earn more money, as the bypass costs highest in the surgery market.

As a matter of fact, an angiography should be done only on the patients who have made up their mind and intend to undergo angioplasty or bypass surgery, to locate the specific portion to be bypassed. Otherwise, the other non-invasive tests, viz. ECG, TMT, thallium etc. are enough to diagnose the disease and continue the treatment with medicines and yoga (changed life style, meditation, exercises, asanas, diet modification, stress management etc.).

5.11 Other Chest Pains and Angina

Sometimes due to resemblance of the symptoms, some other diseases are confused with the heart disease. Whenever the patient feels a little chest pain or pain in the left arm, he/she considers it to be angina. In fear he/she calls the doctor. The following diseases are usually confused with heart disease :

Muscular chest pain : Generally muscular chest pain, if on the left side, is confused with angina. There is every possibility of a thrashing pain (physical blow/contusion in the chest muscles). If the pain subsides on application of Moov/Iodex or by taking a pain killer, it is not angina.

Cervical pain in left or right arm : Cervical spondylosis is also a stress-related disease and induces pain in the chest, shoulders and left or right arm. The pain is constant and is relieved by applying Moov or some pain killer. If it does not subside with a tablet of Sorbitrate, it is not angina, and then cervical X-ray would clear the position.

Gastric pain in chest : Chest pain can also be caused due to gastritis. Gastric pain sometimes moves to the shoulders and any of the arms, and is associated with sweating, choking sensation or breathing discomfort. In most of the cases the gastric pain, due to resemblance of symptoms, is taken as angina. If the patient pinpoints the pain at a specific place in the chest, it is not angina.

If the pain subsides by taking rest or Sorbitrate, it is angina, otherwise not. Before the treatment is started, the diagnosis must be confirmed in order to get the correct treatment.

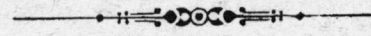

CHAPTER 6

Causative Factors of Coronary Heart Disease

Contents

6.1	Introduction	49
6.2	Non-modifiable risk factors	50
➢	Age, sex, heredity	
6.3	Modifiable risk factors	50

➢ Irregular life-style, stress and mental tension, lack of physical activity, faulty dietary habits, high blood pressure, notorious cholesterol, high blood-cholesterol level, high blood-triglyceride level, high blood-LDL and VLDL levels, high density lipoprotien (HDL) level, diabetes mellitus, obesity, lack of anti-oxidants in diet, isolation, hostility, self-centredness, cynicism, job stress, family stress, greed, sedentary life, smoking and alcohol

Causative Factors of Coronary Heart Disease

6.1 Introduction

Coronary heart disease never develops all of a sudden or in days or weeks like fever, cholera, pneumonia, diarrhoea etc. Heart diseases, however, are the result of a very long period of wrong life-style, e.g. bad food habits, lack of physical activity, excessive cholesterol (fats) and excessive stress. The disease (blockage in coronary arteries) starts from zero and goes on increasing year after year up to the age 30-40. It never gives any indication and one feels quite normal. Only when the blockage crosses 70% and onwards, it is detected and diagnosed in the form of angina or a heart attack.

There are several factors that nourish the origin and development of heart disease. In our professional life, every individual is exposed to those factors, which may be termed risk factors. Some of them are described below

Risk factors : The risk factors responsible for the onset and increased rate of development of heart disease can be broadly grouped under two headings :

(1) The risk factors about which we are unable to do anything, are non-modifiable factors.

(2) The risk factors about which we can do something, can prevent and modify them, i.e. modifiable factors.

We will have to fight against all possible risk factors simultaneously to get the CHD cured.

I. Non-modifiable factors :

1. Age
2. Sex
3. Heredity

II. Modifiable factors :

1. Irregular life-style
2. Stress and mental tension
3. Lack of physical activity
4. Faulty dietary habits
5. High blood-cholesterol level

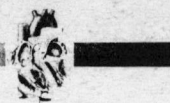

6. High blood-triglyceride level
7. Low blood-HDL and high blood-LDL levels
8. Diabetes mellitus
9. Obesity
10. Lack of anti-oxidants in diet
11. Isolation
12. Hostility
13. Self-centredness
14. Cynicism
15. Job stress
16. Family stess
17. Greed
18. Sedentary life-style
19. Smoking and alcohol

6.2 Non-Modifiable Risk Factors

Age : Heart attack is most frequent during the age of 40-55 years, but it is not uncommon even below this age. Occurrence of heart attack at a younger age is correlated with a strong family history of high blood pressure, diabetes and high blood-cholesterol level as well as heart attacks. Heavy smokers often get heart attacks at ages below 40 years.

Sex : Usually 90% of the heart attacks occur in males. The incidence of heart attacks in females before menopause is markedly less, because the hormone oestrogen protects them. The exact mechanism of this hormonal protection is yet to be clearly understood, but after they attain menopause (at the age of 45 to 50), women are exposed to an equal risk of getting heart attacks as males. This risk is considerably enhanced if the female is a smoker. However, in this moden age the females are under more stress due to increased work load at home as well as at work places. The risk is the same for both under these cirumstances.

Heredity : It has been known for a long time that if several members in a family have heart attack, the chances of their children having heart attack become two-folds at a still younger age. If both the parents have heart disease, the chances of getting a heart attack increase four-folds. Heart attack also occurs in those families where the close relatives have heart attacks at a younger age (age below 40 years). Heart attack in families appears to be both genetic as well as environmental. High blood pressure and diabetes, which cause heart attack, are also known to be genetically determined.

6.3 Modifiable Risk Factors

Irregular life-style : Life-style plays a very important role in the life of every individual and society. It is responsible for the overall development of man. It is the builder of one.'s body and architect of one's mind and character. In this rapidly changing conditions of modern life-style, man has thrown himself away from nature. Our forefathers had developed a foolproof life-style according to the geographical situations and ecological/environmental conditions of India. People were very particular about their physical as well as mental health care. They believed in the dictum: 'early to bed and early to rise'.

People used to get up early in the morning, go for natural compulsions in the jungle, take an early morning walk, do yogic exercises/asanas daily and bathe at the village well in open air, inhaling plenty of oxygen. People were busy in hard work, ladies at home and gents at farms. Ladies also helped men in the fields from time to time. People also used to go to the temples (places of worship) in the morning and evening to enjoy music and dance, attuning their minds towards Gods and Goddesses, which helped them to maintain their mental health and character. The food was cooked on a wooden fire and all the family members took their meals together amid live and coordination. There was never any haste or hurry and everyting was going on very peacefully without any stress or tension and with full contentment.

On the contrary in the modern life-style man is over-loaded and running all the 24 hours of the day. Scarcity of time and space is a great problem. Man has to spend so much time to earn his bread that he finds little time to take meals properly. He is always in a hurry. By chance if the time problem is not there, he finds no space to play, take a walk, do exercises/asanas or to inhale fresh oxygen for a healthy physique and mind.

People have developed wrong food habits too. They believe in rich, fried, fast food and often stale and preserved food instead of preparing it fresh and that too without observing any time schedule, especially in parties. People are fond of watching television (T.V.) sets while taking their meals, not concentrating on the enjoyment the food offers. Watching the scenes of murder, dacoity or violence while taking the meals leaves an adverse effect on the person, especially on children.

In city life of so-called 'developed civilizations', where modern science has put the countries and cities nearer to each other, man has been separated from man, and human life has drifted away from nature. Man has been compelled to live in small flats with his full family and criss-crossed narrow paths full of pollution every day. On the contrary, luxuries and comforts provided by the modern age, instead of adding to the health of the man have rather made him quite lazy. He prefers to operate a T.V. set through a remote control and does not want to take the trouble of going to the set in person to change the volume or the channels. Everybody has become selfish and is running after money and material things, with the greed of possessing more and more. He has forgotten the values of honesty, gentleness, duty and character, which kept the mind calm and heart at peace.

Yogic Cure to Avoid Heart Surgery

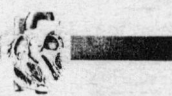

In this modern age of technology, industrialization, overurbanization and fast lifestyle, we are constantly subjected to tremendous stresses and tensions. These in turn produce psychosomatic diseases like hypertension, insomnia, depression and various types of heart ailments. In desperation, people take to drinks and drugs, which of course appear to give a temporary relief, but are dangerous and in fact create more serious troubles.

Stress and mental tension : Stress is considered to be the biggest factor of causing CHD. There is a strong relationship between mental tension/strain and heart disease. People who worry too much get higher blood pressure and have higher incidence of heart attacks. People who are always in a hurry and want to perform too many things in too little a time without any rest are grouped as type 'A' personality of individuals, and have more heart attacks. Heart attack occurs more frequently in a person who has had a sudden economic loss or has lost a close relative.

Excessive stress leads to increase in blood pressure, heart rate, blood sugar, cholesterol and fat deposit. People whose profession involves a lot of mental tension, like businessmen, industrialists, lawyers, doctors, bankers and other high executives, are more prone to heart disease.

Lack of physical activity : With the advancements in technology and rapid economic prosperity, there has been a gradual drop of physical activity in the people. People have left exercise, asanas and related activities; instead they spend their time in non-active pursuits like watching T.V. The body that used to perform much physical activity, now does not get involved physically, denying the muscles any chance to strengthen themselves and the body.

People take a rich diet full of fat, ghee, oil, cream, sweets, etc. In the absence of physical activity, extra calories consumed keep on depositing in the arteries. The previous normal diet has now become quite abnormal. The diet now has to be changed accordingly. If one does not modify one's diet or starts adequate physical activity, the person will have to suffer and pay the penalty thereof, i.e. obesity, hypertension, and heart disease.

Faulty dietary habits : In the prevailing fast-food culture, people not only consume junk food material, totally deprived of necessary nutrients, but also have become habitual of unhygienic and faulty eating styles. We have forgotten the age-old principle of ayurveda of not eating food items of opposite chemical nature at the same time, for example taking ice cream and coffee together. Meals at unscheduled timing very late at night, eating in standing posture etc. have become a status symbol.

All this causes serious problems to our digestive system, leading to several diseases and disorders.

High blood pressure : An ideal blood

pressure in adults ranges between 120-130 mm/Hg systolic (higher) and 80-90 mm/Hg diastolic (lower). If the blood pressure consistently goes beyond 150/100 mm/Hg on two or more occasions, it is called "hypertension", or high blood pressure. It is a very common disease, affecting 20 to 30% adults all over the world. But a majority of the people are not even aware that they are suffering from this disease, because it does not produce any apparent symptoms in a vast majority of them; that is why this disease is called the "silent killer". High blood pressure puts extra strain on the heart and arteries carrying blood supplies to other organs of the body.

Many other diseases are caused by high blood pressure such as heart attack, heart failure, kidney failure, stroke (damage to brain) and damage to eyes. Higher the blood pressure, greater are the chances of getting these diseases. High blood pressure is the main factor for coronary heart disease/heart attack.

Notorious cholesterol : Every heart patient is anxious to know about the cholesterol and how it is responsible for developing the heart disease. How does it play such a role? Cholesterol is a white coloured, wax-like substance mixed in our blood in different forms and running with the flow of blood in the blood stream (blood vessels) throughout the body. In fact it is very essential for the body's systemic functions and we cannot even imagine life without it. But if it exceeds the optimum limits, it becomes dangerous and creates blockage. It gets deposited in coronary arteries, causing or resulting in a short supply of oxygen and nourishment to the heart, leading to a heart attack. In other words, cholesterol is the main culprit of heart disease for vegetarians as well as non-vegetarians.

Cholesterol is produced in the liver. The other sources of cholesterol are the animal products in the form of food, viz. milk, butter, ghee, cheese, ice cream, as well as egg yolk, chicken, fish, meat etc. It also comes from all types of oils including coconut oil. Excess of its associates e.g. triglycerides, LDL and VLDL, are also equally harmful.

High blood-cholesterol level : Nowadays high blood cholesterol is treated to be one of the biggest risk factors of heart disease. Cholesterol is one of the fats found in our blood in combination with proteins. These combinations are called lipoproteins. There is a strong relationship between blood-cholesterol and heart attacks. The people whose blood-cholesterol level exceeds 220 mg/100 ml are prone to get more heart attacks than those having a lower level. The blood-cholesterol level is higher also in people whose diet is rich in cholesterol and saturated fats like cream, butter, ghee, eggs, chicken or meat.

However, unsaturated fatty acids found in various oils like corn oil, mustard oil and soyabean oil have less cholesterol, which help reduce the incidence of heart attacks. Most people maintain a fairly constant level of cholesterol in the blood stream. However, this level may rise with age, dietary habits, lack of physical activity, stress and anxiety. The cholesterol levels in blood can be lowered by taking a low-fat vegetarian diet, reuglar

Yogic Cure to Avoid Heart Surgery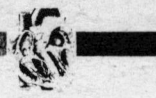

yogic physical exercise, morning walk, and avoiding obesity, stress and smoking.

High blood-triglyceride level : The other fat is triglycerides, which is also a major cause of heart disease. Cholesterol and triglycerides have long been associated with premature coronary heart disease. The dietary fat is broken down by digestive enzymes in the intestines to form free cholesterol fatty acids, mono and diglycerides, which after absorption combine to form triglycerides. Cholesterol and triglycerides are carried in the blood by special proteins, called lipoproteins. There is a correlation between high triglycerides level and coronary artery disease. The ideal level of triglycerides is 60 to 150 mg/dl.

A low-calorie diet, avoiding smoking and restricted or limited use of alcohol are advised for its prevention.

Some oil manufacturing companies nowadays are giving publicity to their products that their oil is hydrogenated has, less triglycerides or is free of triglycerides and hence is beneficial in reducing heart disease. Such advertisements are confusing. In fact all oils have cholesterol/triglycerides and are harmful. They are equally liable for deposits in the arteries, resulting in heart disease.

High blood LDL and VLDL levels : Low-density lipoproteins (LDL), very low-density lipoproteins (VLDL) and cholesterol are responsible for the increased risk of heart disease, because of their deposition in coronary arteries. Hence they are labelled as bad cholesterol. LDL and VLDL carry the fat made in the liver along with cholesterol to the cells of the body, where it harms. The normal level of LDL is 120 mg per 100 ml and of VLDL is 25 mg per 100 ml blood.

The incidence of coronary artery disease can be modified significantly by lowering the cholesterol level, especially the LDL and VLDL components of cholesterol, by diet modification, regular physical exercise and yogic life-style.

High-density lipoprotein (HDL) low level : High-density lipoprotein (HDL) has the opposite effect and protects the coronary arteries. Hence it is called good cholesterol. This is the only cholesterol which we would like you to increase. HDL picks up the excess cholesterol circulating in the blood and carries it back to the liver, to be expelled from the body. If one does very hard work or extra-ordinary work such as continuous travelling or working during son's/daughter's marriage, his/her HDL cholesterol level goes down and a complete rest for a week or so restores the HDL level. The normal level of HDL is 40 mg per 100 ml blood.

Do's and Don't's : To keep the cholesterol, LDL, VLDL and triglycerides at an ideal level and to increase the HDL level, keep the following points on your finger tips :

1. Cut down full-cream milk and dairy products; instead include plenty of vegetables, fruits and whole-grain cereals.

Causative Factors of CHD

2. Other dietary choices for vegetarians are soyabean and various pulses. They have the ability to bring it down through their fibre content. The soluble fibre and cholesterol bind together and are eliminated from the body.

3. The non-vegetarians may follow a diet free from eggs, fish, chicken and mutton. They should try to adopt vegetarian diet as far as possible.

4. Do not forget to cut down the saturated fats found in hydrogenated oils like dalda and butter. These fats increase the LDL level. Polysaturated fats like sunflower, olive, mustard seeds and flax seeds are comparatively less harmful.

5. Coffee and full-cream milk must be substituted with soyamilk.

6. Foods like raw onions, almonds, walnuts and red wine (in small amount), help in increasing the HDL level.

7. Eating three or four garlic cloves daily is benefecial in lowering the blood- cholesterol level.

8. A total cholesterol reading of 180-200 ml/dl (milligram per decilitre) is ideal, 210 to 230 mg/dl is border line and higher level is risky.

9. Calorie-restricted (1200 -1300 calories per day) diet with a variety of foods leads to a healthy life.

10. The key for keeping all cholesterols within safe limits followed with yogic exercises and a correct diet is a disciplined life.

Diabetes mellitus : The normal optimum level of blood sugar in the fasting state is 80-120 mg/dl and after taking meals 160-200 mg/dl. If the fasting level of blood sugar is more than 120 mg/dl or after meals more than 160 mg/dl, it is called the state of diabetes or high blood sugar. In diabetic patients, sugar can be detected in the urine also. Patients with diabetes have a higher prevalence of heart attack. They are usually obese and have high blood pressure and high blood cholesterol, all responsible for the occurrence of attacks.

The symptoms of diabetes include increased thirst, increased urination and weight loss. Morning and evening walks are the best preventive measures for diabetics.

Obesity : If the weight of a person is more than the upper limit of weight for his or her age and height, one is called obese or a fat person (Annexure1). People who eat too much fat and do not do any exercise or physical activity become obese. Such individuals have higher chances of getting high blood pressure, diabetes and heart attacks.

Obese people generally remain inactive. They are often the objects of fun or taunting. Therefore, they tend to develop excesssive mental tension, resulting in hypertension and heart attack. The chances of getting attacks are increased by 15 times in obese people compared with lean and thin ones. Obesity can be prevented by eating low-calorie food, avoiding fats and too much sugar, and performing regular yogic exercises.

Lack of anti-oxidants in diet : There is a group of supernutrients, which are the precursors to vitamin 'A' (beta-carotene), vitamin 'C' (ascorbic acid) and vitamin 'E' (tocopherol). These nutrients together form a powerful alliance to protect the body from many diseases and also forestall the ageing process. These vitamins are present in many types of food and occur naturally in fruits and vegetables. The drugs, in comparison, are less effective and have side-effects too.

The body's use of oxygen derived from food as a fuel for the body processes is remarkable. Oxygen is moved around the body in the blood stream to feed living cells, which prevent heart disease. This process is called oxidation. Therefore, a balanced diet with sufficient amount of anti-oxidants in the form of vitamins A, C and E along with moderate exercise and pranayama shall provide sufficient amount of fuel and oxygen to every cell and system of the body, which shall keep both the body and mind healthy and at the same time will reduce the ageing process, besides subsiding the coronary artery disease.

Isolation : Isolation is a major cause of coronary heart disease, skin diseases, and even cancer. Isolation is not merely loneliness or solitude, it is a sense of aloofness, unconnectedness, even alienation. It is an emotional condition, and an acute feeling that a person is left all alone, high and dry in almost all situations that matter to him or have a meaning of his existence. Often retirement leads to this condition. For instance, a retired executive, who has enjoyed power once, feels that now he is out of office and people have ceased to respect him. A young man striving to build his career may have a stern boss or uncooperative and hostile colleagues to deal with; and is compelled to continue in his job, suppressing his anger, and thus feels helpless. A talented person might feel that his talent is not recognised and he is not appreciated, and thus feels quite bitter.

Even domestic discord and tension might make one feel rather isolated in one's own home in the midst of near and dear ones. A spouse might feel isolated when he/she feels neglected by the other, who might be over-occupied and lost in his or her pursuits. Loss of spouse after a long and happy married life creates a void and is a major risk factor resulting in heart attack or even cancer during the first year of bereavement. A child might feel isolated, when parents are too busy to give attention and care, particularly if the child has a problem and needs support.

Isolation is painful, as it saps (destroys) the real joy of living. Isolation often breeds hostility, cynicism, self-centredness, a sense of guilt and gloom, which leads to serious illness, particularly coronary heart disease. It has a very adverse effect on the body, specially on the immune system and blood chemistry. The isolated individual may take to alcohol, tobacco chewing and smoking, which might further aggravate the risk of coronary heart disease.

Hostility : The dictionary meaning of hostility is "revengeful attitude". In its larger sense it includes extreme intolerance, aggressive behaviour, unreasonable anger and dislike for an individual. Normally, we consider tolerance as a virtue, but in reality if you tolerate half-heartedly with an inner dislike, it is nothing but suppressed anger, and it has the same effect as anger on the heart. Hostility can be due to the lack of parental care during childhood, which results in a sense of insecurity and injustice at home or at school from colleagues and teachers. Children who have experienced such injustice during childhood feel very bitter about everything, and develop hostility against the whole world on the slightest pretext. Hostility breeds extremely irritable temper and self-centredness with a cynical attitude towards everything and everyone. With this temperament one looks at everyone with contempt and feels isolated.

Self-centredness : Self-centredness arises out of a sense of utter insecurity. When an individual feels very insecure, he seeks self-interest without the least concern for others. Even at the prospect of harming others he sticks to self-interest. One becomes so very egocentric that it tends to narrow not only one's outlook on life but also adversely affects the arteries.

Cynicism : When an individual finds fault with everything good or bad, and has lost all faith in goodness of life, he becomes contemptuously cynical; and this attitude again, according to Dr Dean Ornish, poisons the heart.

Job stress : Stress due to the insecurity of job, a sense of injustice, constant tussle with the boss, non-cooperation of colleagues, ambition to rise above everyone else in a short time, jealousy and vicious competition are the apparent causes of heart attack amongst the young persons. Problems in business, financial, managerial and labour matters cause great stress.

A 35-year-old young employee of the State Bank of India, who had come under the influence of Shri Aurobindo and Mother was living a contented, healthy life. At an examination conducted by the employer for promotion, a colleague with much less competence got the promotion and he was left out. For nearly 3 years he remained stressed under the sense of severe injustice and felt isolated. He was struck with a coronary affliction. After angiography he was even advised bypass surgery. Such a sense of dissatisfaction with the whole world probably results in coronary heart disease.

Family stress : An unexpected financial crisis, a long-drawn expensive illness, marital problems, shocking catastrophic family events and conflicts with children are usually the causes of family stress, which may also result in coronary heart disease in the individuals who are prone to it on other scores.

Greed : We live in a socio-economic set up where the whole day one works hard at an inhuman speed of physical and intellectual operations. The way we move, we go on collecting things at a material level, knowledge on the intellectual level, and experience on the sensual and physical level. With every experience and achievement, we build up our ego and create an enclosure around us. In that enclosure we feel secure and live a secluded and isolated life from our real self because of the sense of possession. Greed is a very common human trait. If something benefits an individual, he would naturally like to have more of it, whether name, fame, money, rare or ancient articles, books, paintings and other worldly goods. There is a thin line between greed and ambition. Even in good pursuits like spreading humanitarian ideas, such as usefulness of yoga in everyday life, one may overstep.

Sedentary life : Sedentary life-style or tendency of not doing any physical work is also one of the important factors for heart disease. Several studies have shown that people who do more of desk jobs, such as clerks, officers, doctors, lawyers, businessmen etc., get more heart attacks than those whose professions require more of physical exertion, e.g. farmers, labourers, bus conductors etc. People who have sedentary life-styles do not do regular physical exercise and are over-weight. With inadequate functioning of their lungs and circulation they can also develop various joint and bone disorders. Regular physical exercise not only prevents diseases like joint pains, hypertension and heart attacks but also keeps a person more fit, efficient, active and zealous. His lungs are stronger, the joints are healthy and flexible and his face and skin remain young.

Therefore, exercise not only adds years to life but also life to years.

Smoking and alcohol : Smoking of cigarettes, bidis and taking tobacco in any form, i.e. zarda, gutka, khaini etc., are dangerous for causing the development of diseases like heart attack, cancer of the lungs, bronchitis, ulcers, narrowing of arteries etc. Several scientific studies have shown that heart attack occurs with increased frequency in smokers. The disease is most frequent in heavy smokers and occurs at much younger age. The death rate due to heart attacks is also higher in smokers. The risk of heart attacks and other diseases diminishes if one stops smoking. Even smoking one cigarette does considerable harm to the body. The risk of getting a heart attack is increased by at least 4-folds in people who smoke 15 cigarettes or more a day.

Alcohol is also equally a risk factor for coronary heart disease. It increases triglyceride level and contributes to fat and neurological damage. Wine or alcohol often cause disputes and spoil harmonious relations in the family, which ultimately creates stress and leads to blockage in the arteries.

Section 3

Stress and Coronary Heart Disease

CHAPTER 7

Stress

Contents

7.1	Introduction	63
7.2	What is stress?	63
7.3	Salient factors of overload stress	64

➢ Work overload, time overload, requirement overload, information overload, sickness overload

7.4	Seven sectors of life synthesis	67

➢ Work and profession, money, health, family, love and affection, social life, spiritual atmosphere

7.5	Stress and psychosomatic diseases	68
7.6	Salient symptoms of excessive stress	69

➢ Physical symptoms, behavioural symptoms, emotional symptoms, cognitive symptoms, physiological symptoms

Stress

7.1 Introduction

Every human being has always been in constant search of happiness, inner peace, love and affection. To achieve this, people continue to pursue money and power, and even after achieving it if they are uncontented, unhappy and have an unquenchable thirst for more and more, which amounts to tremendous stress-that affects their life and health adversely, it may lead to coronary heart diseases .

The great poet and philosopher Lord MacEnzie says :

"Luxury makes a man so soft that,
It is hard to please him and easy to trouble him;
So that his pleasure at last becomes his burdon .
Luxury is a nice master, but hard to be pleased".

7.2 What is Stress?

Stress is a univeral word, which is being used by everyone, everywhere. A clear-cut definition has not yet been evolved. However, you may also try to define stress. Some definitions, though, are tried here.

Medical : Medical science describes stress as a specific response of the body to all non-specific demands, be it physical or psychological, threatened or actual. The responses are the secretions of ACTH (adrenocorticotropic hormone) and cortisol. These are two stress-induced hormones. There are two other stress-stimulated secretions of hormones, i.e. adrenaline and non-adrenaline.

Practical : A more practical definition of stress may be put as, "When the problems presented by everyday routine life exceed our resources for coping with them, we feel stress". But we must remember that stress cannot be imposed solely by external demands created by problems, but can also be generated from within, that is internally by our hopes, fears, expectations and beliefs.

Stress is the biggest problem in the human

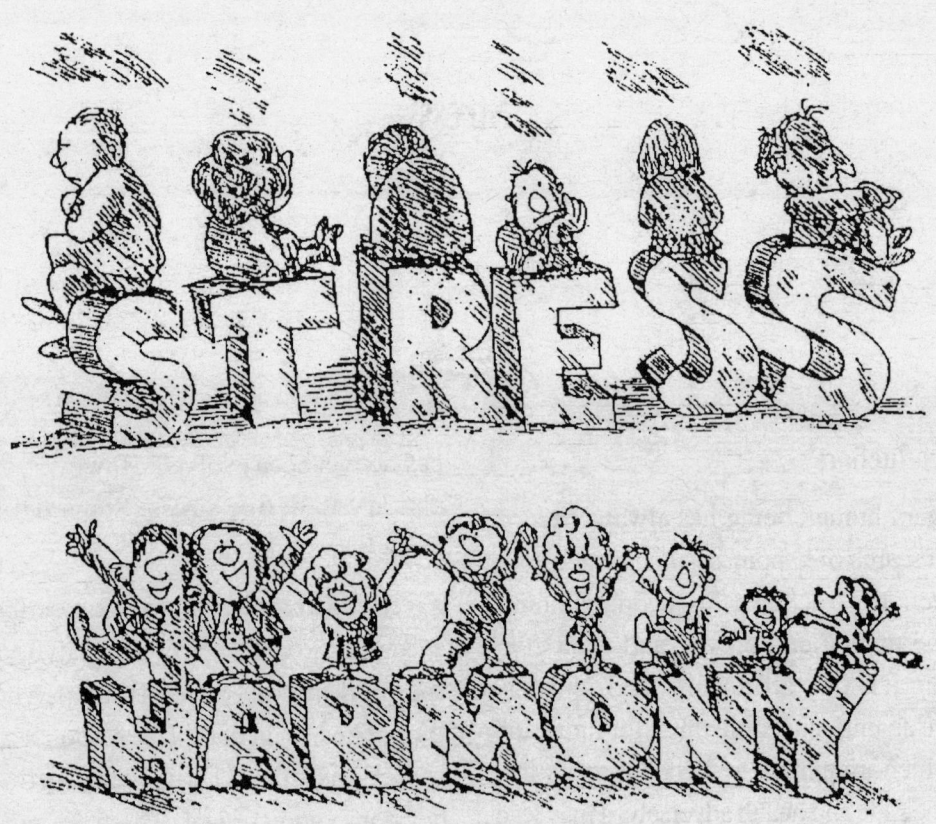

Fig. 7.1 Stress versus harmony

mind. Personality of an individual under stress is cast down in his spirit, or we can say that stress defines the personality of a man (Fig.7.1).

Now the question arises : Is it possible to have money and power on one hand and the good qualities of life, i.e. efficiency, friendship, peace and happiness, on the other? Here in this section some processes are described in a step-wise manner or how we can achieve a perfect equilibrium between the demands and stress of life without unduly taxing our normal daily routine. In other words, we can call it the science and art of living or the yogic life style. The same is required to be adopted for a perfectly balanced happy life.

7.3 Salient Factors of Overload Stress

A dynamic individual is a typically stressed person. In routine he involves himself in hurry for work, skipping breakfast or gobbling down an inadequate amount of food, working right through lunch and till late in the evenings, a few drinks followed by a high fat, spicy dinner with business associates or clients. He returns home late at night to retire for the day, only to repeat this exhausting routine the next day. Perhaps he forgets that he is spending so much amount of time to earn his bread that no time is left for him to eat that bread. Improper planning, misarranged daily routine, lack of physical activity, relaxation and rest to the body and mind are obviously missing from the daily routine of common individuals. The overload problems being faced by a person are :

1. Work overload
2. Time overload
3. Requirement overload
4. Information overload
5. Sickness overload

Work overload : In ancient times, the type of work was neither so complicated nor so excessive. Everything was easy going. Only one member was to earn and the whole family could be fed comfortably. In the modern life-style, every member of the family has to earn and even then the returns are insufficient to meet the requirements.

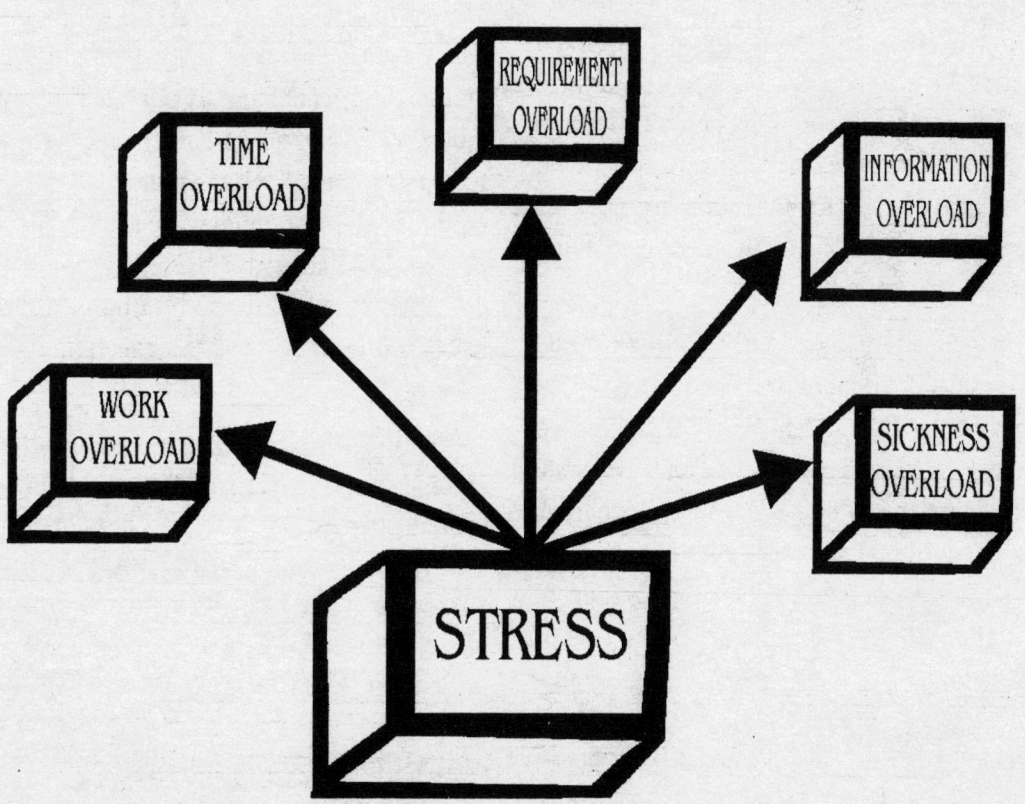

Fig.7.2 Five overload stress components

Yogic Cure to Avoid Heart Surgery

T.V., car, water, electricity, telephone, preparation of food, learning computer, reading, writing, attending to vistors are additonal works which lead to stress. The family is under work stress due to increased work load at home and at work places and thus they have to face the same risks.

Time overload : In ancient and recent past there used to be plenty of work with individuals, but everything was being performed very beautifully and with full patience. There was no hurry any where. Now even the school-going children are to leave home at a fixed time. Earning members have to reach office at a fixed time. We are time bound at each and every step. In the office weekly, monthly, quarterly returns are to be filled in a prescribed time period. If you are late by a couple of minutes, you will miss your bus and will have to wait for the next bus, leading to stress.

Requirement overload : Requirements now-a-days have increased considerably and excessively. My grand-father was having two pairs of dhoti-kurta, my father had four-five pairs, I have 15 pairs of shirts and trousers, whereas my son requires 50 pairs, and there is need to tax the brain about the requirments of my grandson. Even after having more than hundred sets of clothes, he always feels shortage of garments. Whenever family members see flats, cars, watches, dresses, air conditioners, sarees, kitchen wares or any new item anywhere, they feel their requirment accordingly. This is a never- ending process and as a result we have to work more, which needs more time, ultimately leading to requirement overlaod stress.

Information overload : There are plenty of sources now-a-days to cause information overload. T.V., radio, newspaper, magazines, books etc. offer plenty of varied information, entertainment or even gossips. Advertisements through hoarding and pamphlets are very common. Some news-papers contain 50 pages or more, publishing advertisements about films, daily-necessity goods, health aids, health clinics, electrical appliances, educational centres, banquet halls, travel agencies, banking, railway and government tenders, political movements, industrial developments, parliament proceedings, foreign policies, UNO matters, elections, pay commissions, minimum wage act, religious and political programmes/meetings, games and so on. All this is enough to bombard our mind, causing infomation overload, as if our brain is a "sarai".

Sickness overload : Sickness, obviously, has increased sufficiently now-a-days and is growing day by day. It is very common in every family that some of the members are always suffering from one or the other acute or chronic disease, i.e. cough, asthma, diabetes, arthritis or B.P. This is a natural phenomenon, particularly in the old age, and we cannot escape this condition. One should take the situation patiently, peacefully, lovingly and smilingly.

7.4 Seven Sectors of Life Synthesis

Another important factor for increasing the stress is the improper balancing of seven sectors of life synthesis. Those who fail to maintain the co-ordinaton among these sectors, have to face the state of stress tremendously. These are :

less money for it, viz. principal of a college, director or managing director. But some prefer to earn more money whatever the status may be. What is important is that one must love his work or profession.

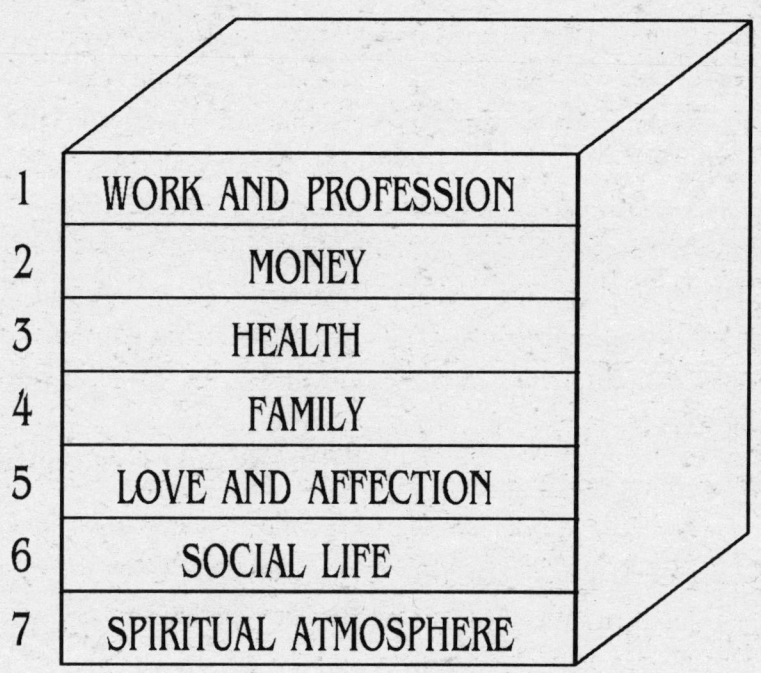

Fig. 7.3 Seven sectors of life synthesis

Work and profession : Assess yourself whether you are satisfied with your work or profession. You like it or dislike it. If one does not like his work, stress becomes high. Some prefer to become a boss, with many people working under them even though they might get

Money : Money sector does not mean that your earnings are in lakhs or crores. It does not matter if it is less, but your income and expenditure should be balanced. Your routine expenditure must not exceed your earnings; only then your money sector is strong.

Health : Health is also a matter of great concern in the modern society. Everybody has some health problem, which leads to stress. One should be educated on proper habits, yogic exercises/asanas and meditation. Your health should be perfect. Try to live happily and keep your body fit.

Family : Family sector is also a very important sector. Some people remain happy at their work place, but immediately on entering their home they become stressful, either due to their wife, father, son or daugther-in-law. If all members in the family live in coordination and have love for each other as well as for the head of the family, home is heaven. Divorces and separations have now-a-days become a common phenomenon. Every member should be careful for the likes and dislikes of others too.

Love and affection : Your family members respect and love you. But do you too have a sense of love and sacrifice for them or you have only expectations from them? Whether your sons/daughters give you respect or are waiting for your early last breath? This sector can be strengthened by sacrifice and love for others. If you feel that your family members will stand by you during a crisis, your love sector is strong.

Social life : Are you and your family members well connected with the society? Do they participate in others' occasions of sorrow and happiness? Please remember, if you do not participate in such social activities, nobody will care for you when you are in need. Many tasks are such which can be performed only with the help of society and not with money, viz. admission of a child in a school or college or to find a good match for your son or daughter. You will feel helpless when money fails to meet such needs.

Spiritual atmosphere : Another important factor that is ignored mostly by people is spiritual faith, attitude and atmosphere. If you are committing any act not permitted by the society or by the law, your conscience would scold you, leaving you unhappy and under stress. Have you enough faith in God? If you are dishonest anywhere, you cannot lead a stress-free life. Achievements through unfair means can never provide you the real peace or happiness.

7.5 Stress and Psychosomatic Diseases

Modern science, till 2 decades back, did not attribute stress to be the cause of diseases. Hypertension, heart disease, peptic ulcer, cervical spondylosis etc. are very common in highly placed executives, though it is not generally found in low- earning native villagers, farmers or labourers. This interesting finding can only be explained on the basis of severe stress. In the last few decades a series of epidemiological studies and observations have proved that some very common diseases are the direct result of excessive stress. They are now grouped as **psychosomatic diseases.**

Stress-induced common diseases :
1. High blood pressure
2. Angina, chest pain
3. Heart attack
4. Tension, headache, migraine
5. Backache/shoulder ache/body ache
6. Cervical spondylosis
7. Asthma/bronchial asthma
8. Allergy
9. Chronic fatigue
10. Anxiety state, depression
11. Insomnia/sleeplessness
12. Phobia/psychosis/neurosis
13. Irritable bowel syndrome (IBS)
14. Peptic ulcer

CHD is the most common disease found in people suffering from stress.

7.6 Salient Symptoms of Excessive Stress

Physical symptoms :
1. Tense muscles : shoulderache, backache
2. Irregular breathing
3. Dry mouth
4. Sweating palms
5. Cold fingers
6. Shaky hands
7. Frequent urination

Behavioural symptoms :
1. Smoking : Consumption of cigarettes increased
2. Tobacco : Consumption of gutka etc. increased
3. Stimulant intake : Repeated drinking of tea and coffee
4. Alcohol : Consumption of alcohol and its doses increased
5. Habit of nail biting, knee jingling, finger bending, hair pulling
6. Obsessive/compulsive behaviour : To check things (lock etc.) repeatedly
7. Social withdrawal : Uninterested response to others' talks/wishes
8. Uninterested look : No attention towards self
9. Upset style of living

Emotional symptoms :
1. Irritability
2. Short temper
3. Undue haste
4. State of anxiety
5. Feeling of depression
6. Feeling of insecurity, desire for suicide or killing
7. Undue aggression : Trying to struggle for no reason
8. Sleeplessness
9. Bad dreams
10. Tendency of not taking any type of responsibility

Yogic Cure to Avoid Heart Surgery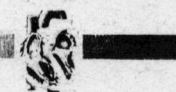

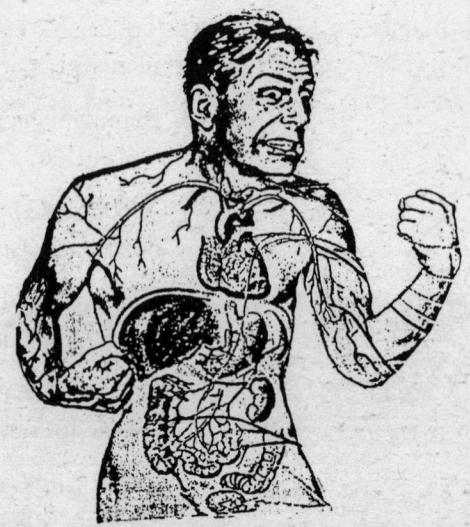

Fig. 7.4 A man under the state of acute stress

Congnitive symptoms :

1. Loss of sense of humour
2. Loss of memory
3. Forgetfulness
4. Loss of common sense
5. Loss of clarity in thinking
6. Indecisiveness
7. Undue fear
8. Lack of creativity.

Physiological symptoms :

1. Heart rate increases
2. Blood pressure increases
3. Muscle tension increases : Distribution of excessive blood to voluntary muscles
4. Galvanic skin resistance (G.S.R.) decreases
5. Respiratory rate increases
6. Oxygen consumption increases
7. Spasm of arteries
8. Sweating
9. Dilation of bronchial tube
10. Decreased urine production
11. Serum cortisol increases
12. Blood sugar increases
13. Serum catecholamines increase
14. Serum cholesterol increases

All these symptoms occurring in combination lead to coronary heart diseases, of mild to severe degree, proving that stress is one of the major factors producing CHD.

CHAPTER 8

Stress Management

Contents

8.1	Introduction	73
8.2	Ideal stress	73
8.3	Excessive stress	73
8.4	Production of stress	73
	➢ Internal stressers, external stressers, environmental stressers	
8.5	Keys to cope with stress	74
	➢ Recognition and identification of stress, avoiding and forgetting the incidences, minor modification in routine matters to cope with stress	
8.6	Strategies for stress management	75
	➢ When you are angry, when anger has cooled down but chronic stress of anger is present, skill of communication, anuvrat (development of moral values), anekant (theory of multiple views or non-absolutism), anupreksha (development of will power)	
8.7	Skill of time management	77
8.8	Jotting down exercises	78
8.9	Meditation	79
8.10	Kayotsarga (self-relaxation)	79

Stress Management

8.1 Introduction

No doubt, stress is the biggest factor in causing coronary heart disease, but at the same time it is quite essential for life. Without stress you cannot achieve any thing of significance in society and perform any of your duties and responsibilities with vigour or stand for your rights. Since no device has yet been invented to measure stress, we can divide the people into two major categories in respect of stress, i.e. (i) ideal stress and (ii) excessive stress.

8.2 Ideal Stress

Stress, as obvious, is essential to perform any work or achieve the goal of life, otherwise one would become lazy, incompetent, irresponsible and frustrated. With such a stress to achieve your goal, you put forth energy in your work and plan for its success. With a pint of stress under your arm-pit, you may be able to handle life situations successfully. You should love your work or profession and perform it with full contentment and without any agitation. You should respect others and maintain a harmonious relation with your neighbours, colleagues, subordinates, seniors and anyone who comes into your contact. For all this, some stress is necessary and that stress is called `ideal stress'. Persons enjoying such a stress come under `Type B' category.

8.3 Excessive Stress

Some people treat themselves as successful in life, but they are unaware that they remain under excessive stress. They generally have too much work to do and multiple problems to solve before them every time. Usually they are short of time, restless, impatient and suffer from fatigue. They feel exhausted on returning home late at night and loaded with high stress, frustration and discontentment in their mind. They cannot sleep well and usually depend upon sleeping pills. They never feel fresh on getting up in the morning. Such people catch coronary heart disease very easily and come under the category of `Type A' personality.

8.4 Production of Stress

Origin of stress can be derived from three

major sources, i.e. (i) internal stressers, (ii) external stressers and (iii) environmental stressers.

Internal stressers : Internal stressers are the reflections and results of our education, training, tendencies, nature, experiences, attitude, beliefs, hopes and expectations.

External stressers : External stressers are the ones that influence us from outer environment and compel us to react. If we are able to handle them properly, we can overcome these stressers easily and can lead a happy and peaceful life.

Some examples of stress :

At home :

1. Unreasonable desires and expectations.
2. Difference in liking and disliking of husband/ wife and other members of the family.
3. Difference in sleeping patterns, work sharing, rude behaviour from any of the family members.
4. Difference in moral values due to generation gap and similar reasons.
5. Frequent visits of guests and their undesired expectations and demands.

At work place :

1. Difficult boss and imcompetent juniors.
2. Poor administration and lack of skill.
3. Time and work overload, shortage of space.
4. Lack of co-operation and team spirit among colleagues.
5. Uncomfortable chair, poor lighting, ventilation and/or cleanliness.

Environmental Stressers:

1. Pollution and overcrowded cities.
2. Overindustrialization and water/noise pollution.
3. Power and water crisis.
4. Adulterated food and drugs, dishonesty.
5. Excessive dearth and unemployment.
6. Corrupt and incompetent ministers/leaders.
7. Excessively cold or hot weather.

8.5 Keys to Cope with Stress

As stress plays a big role in our daily routine life, the question arises, 'How it is to be faced and solved? Some key points are suggested here.

Recognition and identification of stress : Firstly stress should be recognised and identified regarding location where from it has been originated. It may be due to a difficult boss, notorious junior, a bad neighbour, excessive heat or cold, heavy rains, late trains or buses etc., you can easily pin-point the cause or reason. Sometimes we become unnecessarily stressful by remembering undesired past incidents, which serve no purpose in the present, or fear of future problems which may or may not come. Once you are able to trace and identify the origin of stress, half the stress would be over.

Avoiding and forgetting the incidences

If you are worried about someone's abusive language or indecent behaviour, forget it and try to avoid that person or contact him the minimum. Try to develop the habit of remaining indifferent and overlook the incidents such as winning or losing a test match, railway accidents or plane crashes, dacoity or theft incidents appearing in dailies, different statements given by politicians etc. But it does not mean that you forget unreasonable or undesired happenings. Suppose somebody is not returning a handsome amount he borrowed from you previously, you may fight for its recovery with full strength. But such incidents are very rare.

Minor modifications in routine matters to cope with stress

There are some stresses that can be overcome with slight modification. Suppose lighting in kitchen or room is dim, you may like to replace the bulb with a bulb of higher wattage or a tube or have extra lighting arrangement. If your scooter or car troubles you every day, you may change it, with a better one. If somebody disturbs you or wastes you time, you may easily manage the problem with a slight change in your routine temporarily.

Key

First identify the stress. See if it can be avoided, forgotten or modified. You will definitely find some solution and the stress being experienced will subside.

8.6 Strategies for Stress Management

When you are angry :

1. Do not act in haste; take a deep breath. Count up to 10 or 100. Drink water. Be calm.

2. Think of the positive side of criticism too. If you are wrong, face the fact and listen patiently.

3. Use the anger creatively. Perform some job that needs only your participation, e.g. cleaning an almirah, completion of pending accounts, disposing your income tax file, reading some book of your interest etc.

4. Talk to your close friend or associate, who is a well-wisher and is wise and mature.

5. Learn the art of forgiving.

When anger has cooled down, but chronic stress of anger is present :

1. Try to analyse and reach the root cause of the problem.

2. Train yourself to the art of non-verbal communication.

3. Change your own dialogue if you feel that you had been in the wrong.

4. Understand your critic and respond to him/her appropriately.

5. Make a workable compromise.

Yogic Cure to Avoid Heart Surgery

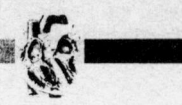

Skill of communication :

The art of communication plays a very important role in avoiding stress for an executive, official or a family man. Half of the family stresses are due to bad skill of communication. Some tips in this regard are given here:

1. Listen properly to the other person who wants to speak. Your posture should be receptive. Everyone desires to be listened to properly.

2. Never criticise directly. Do not insult. Only express your feeling. Speak softly and to the point. For example,

Suppose you come home tired from the office in the evening and ask your wife for a cup of tea. She prepares it and serves it to you okay. You take a sip and find that it has no sugar.

(i) You immediately burst upon her, "You are good for nothing, you cannot even prepare a cup of tea properly". She feels insulted, gets irritated and in turn starts to point out your weak points, and a quarrel starts. It reaches to such an extent that both of you are not on speaking terms for 2-3 days. A high stressful condition.

(ii) On the contrary, you could have smilingly said, "Perhaps you forgot to put sugar in the tea". She would have immediately said, "I am sorry! I'll bring some sugar or shall I prepare fresh tea for you? Please leave this one", and then she would have sat with you in a very good mood and would have served something additional. The environment would have been pleasant. No stress at all.

3. Think over on the discussion. Mentally decide first in which tone and what words you are going to speak, and then speak. As the Baital (ghoul) said to king Vikramaditya:

'Daant oth ekatra kar,

    banh samhare toliye;

Baital kahe Vikram suno,

    jibh samhare boliye.'

(Joining the teeth and lips, weigh while keeping the hands firm. Baital says that listen Vikram, utter a word, only after giving it a prior thought.)

4. Break the spiralling process. Preferably change the topic or say, "Sorry, now let us discuss something else. We will discuss this topic some other time". As the Britishers say, discuss the weather.

5. For regular communication decide the tone of communication. Your speech should be framed in such a style that neither you nor the listener may feel the stress. This will save your energy and provide you pleasantness.

Anuvrat (development of moral values) :

Decline in moral values is a curse to the modern society. Of course every body believes in honesty, truthfulness, non-violence etc., but practically they remain unconcerned. Aruvrat teaches us about development of moral values.

For building a better and ideal personality we should follow Anuvrat principles as specified here.

1. Try to understand that others too have the right of existence.
2. Never become violent. Never try to let down others.
3. Fix limitations of your needs/consumptions.
4. Maintain purity of means.
5. Maintain fearlessness and truthfulness.

Anekant (theory of multiple views or non-absolutism) :

Anekant theory of multiple views or theory of non-absolutism is a Jain philosophy, which preaches us to honour and give due weight to views of other people also. It is not proper to assume : **"Only I am correct and the others are incorrect"**. A single fact or event is bound to be analysed differently by separate individuals. This depends on the factor of an individual's training of moral values and his priorities etc. Suppose a member of your family believes in early to bed and early to rise and he gets up at 5 a.m., whereas you prefer to get up at 7.30 a.m. Both of you are reasonable and correct but both of you will have to adjust mutually. Every person has his own thinking and rights to express his views. **Follow Anekant.** Of course, if you do not agree with the other's view-point, never try to dishonour others intentionally. Try to be co-operative. This will avoid many unnecessary conflicts and help you to preceive the opinion of other people.

Anupreksha (development of will power):

Very often, will power is the key behind a successful executive. Meditation or Kayotsarga is one good tool for developing will power. Sticking to fairness and moral principles makes a significant increment in will power. Every person has unlimited will power, but very often it is not fully explored. Contemplation (Anupreksha) helps in this process immensely.

8.7 Skill of Time Management

1. Are you completely happy with the way you spend your time? we have altogether 24 hours with us in a day. Every individual from the president to a labourer in the world is in the same boat in this regard. And all of them manage their work schedule in the same time frame. How far better you can happily complete all your responsibilities/duties depends upon your **time-management skill.** It is best to decide a long-term plan of your schedule and then check your progress from time to time.

2. An ideal sleep should be of 6-7 hours a day. If you feel tired at noon, take rest for half an hour after lunch.

3. Keep at least 1 or 2 hours a day for your family other than your routine, i.e. bathing, dressing, breakfast etc. Your routine chores should take 2-3 hours a day only and the rest

of the time should be for other things. Try to complete your routine work on week days and relax on holidays. Avoid fixed appointments. Always keep range.

4. Now see your priorities and divide your time for each item accordingly. If you feel that you can complete your task in the time you have, then very good; otherwise shift, divide or pass the whole of it or a part of it to your colleagues or juniors, or refuse to take the additional workload. Re-arrange your priorities.

5. Analyse your time management. You would find that many of us do not actually spend all the time in acutal working, but waste a lot of time in useless affairs.

Some **time-wasting factors** are listed here, for your analysis and action :

   (i) Telephone interruption
   (ii) Meetings/visitors
   (iii) Lack of information
   (iv) Excessive paper work
   (v) Lack of competence, policies, procedures and co-ordination
   (vi) Unclear objectives
   (vii) Failure to set priorities
   (viii) Poor scheduling and poor work division
   (x) Lack of relevant skills
   (xi) Lack of self-discipline

8.8 Jotting Down Exercises

1. Some chronic problems can be solved by jotting down the points in favour or against, analysing all the perspectives and thinking of a possible solution of the problem. You will find the remedies very clear on the written document.

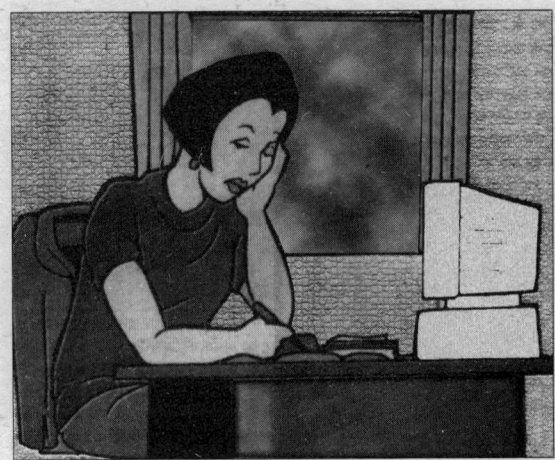

Fig. 8.1 Jotting down exercise

2. Write down how many times you remained under stress during the day. Write the occasions. Now try to solve each by different means as indicated earlier. Using communication skills or by adjustment of internal factors, you can solve those problems. Try some more choices.

3. You will see that this formula works wonders.

8.9 Meditation

1. Yoga says and the doctors also admit that a deep thought by repeated reinforcement affects the psycho-neuro-endocrine as well as psycho-neuro-immune systems and creates the desired changes in the body and mind.

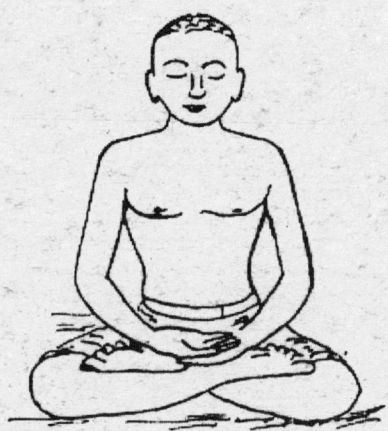

Fig. 8.2 State of Meditation

2. Through meditation a headache can disappear or an enmity can turn into friendship. Anupreksha is a good tool, having immense power to solve any chronic problem. With proper practice of contemplation (Anupreksha), the will power and work efficiency improves gradually.

8.10 Kayotsarga (Self-relaxation) a technique of preksha meditation system

Kayotsarga is a very powerful tool to release any type of stress. A daily session of kayotsarga for 15-20 minutes provides more physical and mantal rest than a sleep of 2 hours.

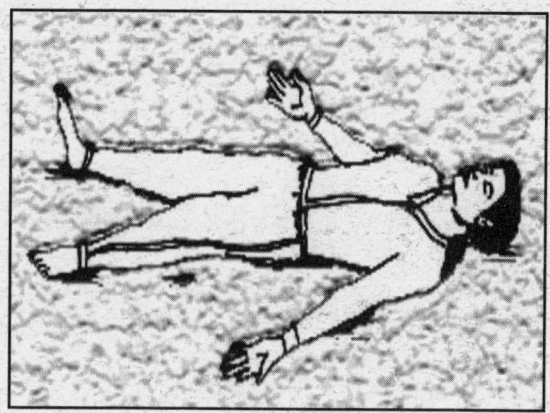

Fig. 8.3 State of Kayotsarga (Self-relexation)

The Kayotsarga keeps the man tension free for the whole day. Its benefits are amplified if added with perception of breathing. Daily practice of kayotsarga is highly recommended.

Section 4

Yogic Management of Coronary Heart Disease

CHAPTER 9

Yoga as a Remedy for Inadequate Modern Drugs in CHD

Contents

9.1	Introduction	85
9.2	Symposium on problems of drug resistance in different diseases	85
9.3	National conference of yoga reasearch and application	86

Yoga as a Remedy for Inadequate Modern Drugs in CHD

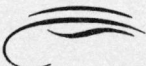

9.1 Introduction

Coronary heart disease is a major cause of death in the modern age. It results from the deposits of cholesterol and fat, which lead to the blockage of arteries, which in turn obstructs the supply of oxygen and blood to the heart muscles. The deficiency of blood and oxygen leads to angina and heart attacks. The basic reasons for these fat deposits are faulty diet (rich in cholesterol and fat), stress, high blood pressure, obesity, lack of physical activity, smoking etc.

Most modern treatments like bypass surgery and angioplasty are, however, useless in the long run for the treatment of coronary disease, in which a steadily increasing number of patients is coming back with the reblockage. The so-called treatment with medicines gives a false sense of relief, and does not reduce the blockage completely. The final result is an exorbitant increase in the number of heart patients and deaths, instead of their decrease.

9.2 Symposium on Problems of Drug Resistance during Different Diseases

In 1997 a symposium was organised by Ranbaxy Science Foundation at National Institute of Immunology, New Delhi. Eminent scientists from different medical institutes gathered there and delivered lectures about "Problem of drug resistance in different diseases". Prof. J.S. Laderberg of Rockefeller University, New York (winner of 1958 Noble Prize in Bacteri Genetics) alarmed the world by declaring that all existing drugs may not be effective in future for treating any disease because microbes are most plastic in changing themselves to adapt to adverse agents. Prof. G. Padmanabham from Indian Institute of Science, Bangalore and Dr P.K. Chakroborti from Tata Memorial Hospital, Mumbai also discussed the alarming situation of drug resistance in malaria. Similarly, Dr P.R. Narayanan, Tuberculosis Research Centre, Chennai; Dr S.E. Hasnain, National Institute of Immunology, New Delhi; and

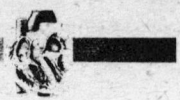

Dr D.N. Pandey from AIIMS, New Delhi also emphasised on the problem of drug resistance in tuberculosis, respiratory and chest diseases. Dr H.S. Adwani from Tata Memorial Hospital, Mumbai also highlighted the problem of drug resistance in cancer.

Prof. Deo from Jaslok Hospital, Mumbai, in response to the above problem of drug resistance, suggested introduction of `Immunotherapy' as an alternative method of treatment. To deal with the above-narrated problems, he stressed upon more researches in the field of improving our own defence system and enhancing the strength of WBC in our blood instead of depending upon drugs. At the end, Prof. J. Shua from Adenberg concluded that the chemotherapies and immunotherapies alone would not be sufficient to tackle this problem. To meet future challanges of emerging drug resistance, we will have to take a decision for more comprehensive approach in the field. Though drugs are important, strengthening of our own body's natural defence system is essential.

Therefore research should be done in this field to enable us to fight against the antigens of all classes. If our body's defence system is strong, we may not need any drugs. Yoga therapy may provide such a strength. To avoid side-effects and adverse reactions of modern drugs, only yoga can come to our rescue.

9.3 National Conference on Yoga Research and Application

Again in February 1998 another National conference in "Yoga research and application" was organised by Central Research Institute of Yoga, New Delhi, where many learned yoga scholars, specialists, doctors, scientists, health workers and philosophers participated. Prof. Madan Mohan from Jawaharlal Nehru Medical Institute, Pondicherry emphasised that our health-care system is woefully inadequate, especially in villages where 75 per cent population of the country lives. Hospitals are over-crowded, under-staffed and starved of funds. Drugs are costly and beyond the reach of common man, besides having many undesirable effects. On the contrary, yoga is inexpensive, easy, scientifically sound and rich in method for improving the health. Shri Anand P. Ashtekar, from Yoga Vidya Niketan, Mumbai discussed about Shat Karmas. The body is the temple of soul and therefore it should be properly maintained. He explained the importance and uses of yogic asanas, kriyas, pranayama, etc. to attain a healthy body and mind.

Dr Ganesh Shankar stated that according to yoga, mental disturbance is a disease and absence of mental disturbance is health. The main aim of yoga therapy is to build up an intergrated personality through a healthy body and healthy mind. Researchers have proved that yogic practices directly influence the body organs to counteract repeated irritations causing stiffness.

They influence the visceral organs and thus cause imbalanced metabolic activity. Pranayama and meditation influence the autonomic nervous system (ANS) by influencing sympathetic and para-sympathetic nerves.

Shri S.D. Bhatnagar from C.R.I.Y., New Delhi pointed out that the present educational system requires intimate knowledge, which could fulfil the need of an individual to live as a harmonious member of the universe. Yoga is a science of education for the formation of character, expansion of intellect and strengthening of mind. Yoga and education are identical processes. The function of yogic education is to guide and coordinate the research activities in the various aspects of yoga, particularly its preventive, protective and curative potential. Dr Ishwar V. Basavardhi from Karnataka University also emphasised and supported the views of Shri Bhatnagar that yoga should be introduced as one of the subjects in colleges and universities for the intergral development of students' personality.

On stress, Prof. S.C. Jain and Prof. B. Talukdar from Maulana Azad Medical College, New Delhi emphasised that it has been incorporated socially and genetically during human evolutionary process. Stress has been a modulating factor for the development and alteration in civilisation and their intellect. It is viewed from its negative impact on human emotional and social behaviour. In biochemical context, stress can be quantified by assessment of free redical-induced destruction of cellular function and integrity. Stress affects ageing and leads to some health disorders like diabetes and hypertension. Simple yogasanas and pranayama techniques provide protection against oxidative stress.

Dr V.S. Vargrecha and Dr H.S. Gaur from Sagar University, Madhya Pradesh emphasised that every second, thousands of stimuli are affecting our body and mind. We are constantly bombarded with external as well as internal influences, which often produce incoherent responses. However, through yogic practices and yogic life-style we can very well improve our resources and ego strength. Thus we can lead a peaceful and stress-free life through yoga.

Dr J.P.N. Mishra from Jain Vishwa Bharti Institute (deemed university), Ladnun in Rajasthan, displayed comparative data of the study on the effect of yogic practices and preksha meditation (kayotsarga and shwas preksha) on the P.G. students appearing for the annual examination. It was aimed to investigate the possible positive response of preksha-yoga in coping with stress caused by the forthcoming annual examinations. Dr Mishra said that the students in the age group 22 to 26 years were included in the study and divided into two groups. The first group was asked to practice kayotsarga and preksha meditation for 45 minutes daily in the morning and evening for 4 weeks, whereas the other group was left to study as usual. The heart rate, B.P. and respiratory rate were recorded at

Yogic Cure to Avoid Heart Surgery

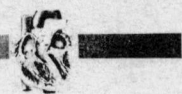

the onset of the study and at the termination of the experiment. The comparative results showed marked reduction in the parameters of Group-I subjects compared with those of Group-II, i.e. better functioning of stress-coping mechanism.

In the end, Swami Dharma Nand, the Director of Adhyatma Sadhana Kendra, Mehrauli, New Delhi, explained his experiences in detail about the preksha- yoga effects, i.e. of asanas, kriyas, pranayama, dhyana and diet management to cope with stress. He emphasised that we should give proper importance to yoga for the welfare of society, mankind, nation and the world. Proper attention to yoga will definitely prove very fruitful.

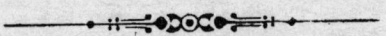

CHAPTER 10

Yoga : Concept, Components and Therapy

Contents

10.1	Introduction	91
10.2	Basis of yoga therapy	91
10.3	Yoga fundamentals	92
10.4	Patanjali's yoga sutra (ashtang yoga)	94

➢ Yama, niyama, asanas, pranayama, pratyahara, dharana, dhyana, samadhi

10.5	Preksha yoga (seven steps)	99

➢ Kayotsarga, antaryatra, shwas preksha, sharir preksha, chaitanya kendra preksha, leshya dhyana, therapeutic thinking through auto-suggestion and contemplation

10.6	Benefits of preksha yoga	103
10.7	Benefits of kayotsarga	103

➢ Relief from tension, freedom from turmoil, revitalisation of the organism, self-awareness, development of aura, development of wisdom

Yoga : Concept, Components and Theraphy

10.1 Introduction

"Yoga is skill in action", states *Bhagavad Gita,* the best known of all the Indian philosophical epics. But this is not intended to mean action in just the narrow sense of physical movement, or simply doing exercises for improving the skill of your body; yoga also comprises techniques that act on your mind and emotions and provides a complete philosophy for living. To achieve this aim, you must develop 'skill' in all aspects of your life. A great Indian teacher of this century, Shri Aurobindo, regarded yoga as a methodical effort towards self-perfection through development of latent potential on the physical, vital, mental, intellectual and spiritual levels. The most fundamental step you can take towards expanding the limits of your consciousness is to gain mastery over your mind.

This is also the key to good health and happiness in today's world. Great advances in medical science over the past century have reduced the incidence of most of the physical diseases that have plagued humanity for centuries. Even better drugs and surgical techniques have led to the eradication of most infectious diseases and the control of many metabolic disorders. Soon even routine genetic interventions may be possible. But these techniques are less effective against the new and even more-common causes of ill health, chronic stress and psychosomatic ailments.

Yoga has a lot to offer. As we approach the 21st century, it gives us the means to complement medical technology with a holistic system of health care that addresses the problems of the mind and spirit as well as those of the body. Patanjali, who wrote the classic text on yoga more than 2000 years ago, described it as "a science of the mind". And it is through teaching you to control your mind, your desires and your reactions to stress that yoga can fundamentally help you.

10.2 Basis of Yoga Therapy

Yoga is fundamentally different from conventional medical practice in its approach to health care. Instead of trying to reduce the cause of disease to a single factor and to correct it using a specific cure, yoga aims to treat illness by improving health on all levels simultaneously and by restoring inner harmony.

Ill health occurs when the total balance of perfect health is disturbed. A bad day at work may make you irritable, exhausted increase your stress reactions and may make your muscles tense and often dissipate your energy levels, leading to chronic fatigue.

For this reason, yoga contains elements that address the problem at every level : **asanas** that relax and tone your muscles and massage your internal organs; **pranayama** that slows breathing and regulates the flow of prana; **kayotsarga, (relaxation)** and **meditation** that act to calm your mind and emotion culturing to heal your spirit. Just as negative influences spread disruption, positive action has repercussions as well. The different types of yoga practices augment each other and are more effective when done together. When you do the **asanas** and stretch your muscles, muscular tension is released and you are able to relax better. Likewise, when you relax the mind and release the suppressed emotions, you tend to become less tense on the physical and mental levels. Every element of yoga brings benefits throughout, and it also amplifies the effect of other types of practices.

This is the essence of yoga therapy, i.e. it acts both as a preventive and as a curative measure. Daily practice of a complete yoga session can restore your natural balance and harmony, bringing positive good health to all parts of your life—physical, mental and spiritual.

10.3 Yoga Fundamentals

Yoga is a philosophical doctrine developed in India by about 500 B.C., based on moral principles, restraint ascetic and meditation techniques and a special type of physical training called hath yoga, which involves control of postures and respiration.

Yoga has been derived from the sanskrit word `yuj', meaning to join, to bind, to attatch or to bring in contact a true union of atma (soul) with Paramatma (the Almighty). It also means to concentrate on a specific point or a specific thought with full and combined attention of mind as well as of body.

In the modern context, yoga may be considered to constitute the most important sector of knowledge, because it is needed by all and can be cultivated according to the inclination and capacity by anyone and of any age, without any limitation of nationality, colour, creed, sex etc. Yoga is generally understood to be concerned with the union or intergration of the following pairs :

— Science and spirituality

— Knowledge and wisdom

— Individual consciousness and universal consciousness

— Individual self and the all pervading spirit

— Man and God

Definition of yoga : Maharshi Patanjali's quotation 'योगश्चित्त वृत्ति निरोधः' ;Yogash chitt vritti nirodhah) is very famous to describe Yoga. "Yoga is the state of nirodha (cessation) of all vritties (fluctuations) in

Yoga: Concept, Components and Therapy

chitta (the psychic, the mental being or the inner instrument of cognition and consciousness)".

(*Yoga-Sutras* - 1, 2, 3)

Lord Krishna in **Bhagwad Gita** describes yoga as 'योगष: कर्मेसु कोशलं' (Yogash karmasu kaushalam), that is to act without desire or greed for result and to maintain an equilibrium between success and failure.

It has further been mentioned : "Let this be known by the name of yoga. The viyoga (disconnection) from samayoga (firm union) with dukha (sorrow or pain), wherein the chitta (mental being) restrained by yoga-seva (yogic practices) comes to rest, wherein one beholds the Cosmic Self through his individual self and rejoices in the Cosmic Self, wherein one experiences that supreme bliss that can be grasped by the buddhi (pure intellect), but is beyond the reach of the senses, wherein established one does not deviate from Truth, on gaining which one cannot conceive of any greater gain than that and wherein the anchored one is not shaken even by the heaviest dukha (sorrow or pain)."

— *Bhagwad Gita*, VI- 23

Jain Acharya Umaswati says about yoga : 'कायवाडमन: कर्म योग:' (Kaya wang manah karm yogah), i.e. the collective function of body, speech and mind is yoga.

— Acharya Umaswati

Sri Aurobindo says about yoga that man is only a transitional being, living in mental consciousness, but with the possibility of acquiring a new consciousness, the Truth consciousness, and capable of living a life perfectly harmonious, good and beautiful, happy and fully conscious. During his whole life, Sri Aurobindo devoted all his time to establish this consciousness in himself and to help those gathered around him to realise it. He called it collective yoga, and integrated yoga, cosmic yoga and spiritual yoga not for individual salvation but for the entire humanity, to be converted into a **super-humanity.**

— Patheya P-II,

Swami Sivananda says that yoga is integration and harmony between thoughts, words and deeds, or integration between head, heart and hands.

— Swami Sivananda

"Yoga is a system of living with a sense of science of the realization of ultimate values and altruistic mission of life. Yoga evolves a harmonious order in mind, matter and man."

— Swami Satyananda Saraswati

Yoga may also be defined as the science of consciousness, the science of creativity, the science of personality development, the science of self and the science of body and mind. Yoga is always concerned with three intergrated components of ourself—body, mind and consciousness. It is, in fact, an augmentation of facts and life-knowledge gained from experience concerning the fudamental importance of a constant state of balance.

Yogic Cure to Avoid Heart Surgery

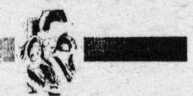

Maharshi Patanjali's *Yoga Sutra (Ashtang Yoga)* **500 B.C. :** Maharshi Patanjali, the authority on Yoga, studied deeply the total yoga in Vedas, Upanishads, Gita and through the Bodh, Mahavira, Charak and other schools, and converted the mystical thoughts of yoga (theory and practice) delveoped by that time, into a systematic order of philosophy, by giving it a proper shape of technique according to Indian traditions in *Ashtang Sutra*. This system is very comprehensive and is under the reach of a common man.

10.4 Patanjali's Yoga Sutra (Ashtang Yoga)

EIGHT STEPS OF YOGA

Patanjali's yoga comprises eight steps, which can be grouped under 3 heads, as follows :

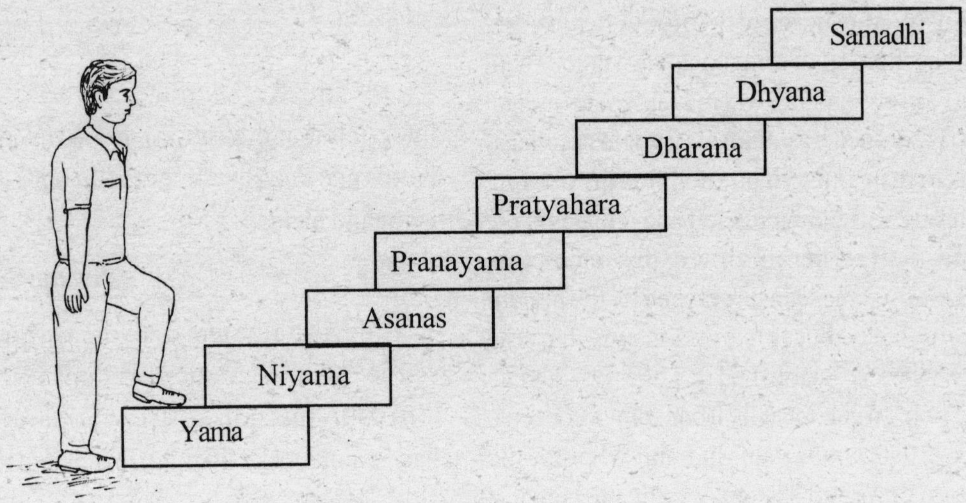

1. Yama
2. Niyama   } Ethical practice

3. Asanas
4. Pranayama
5. Pratyahara   } External yoga

6. Dharana
7. Dhyana
8. Samadhi   } Internal meditation

Yama

It consists of five rules :

1. **Satya (truthfulness) :** Mahatama Gandhi said, 'Truth is God and God is truth'. One should be fair and true in all speech, actions and even in thoughts and conduct. Untruthfulness will lead one away from his/her mission.

2. **Ahimsa (non-violence) :** Not to harm any living being even vegetation (vanaspati) by way of speech or action in any way (not only in outward action but also in thoughts) is true ahimsa. This creates an atmosphere of harmony (harmonious relations) and a sense of brotherhood among people and keeps them away from any type of hatred and ego, besides creating a state of purity of mind, which is an essential factor to achieve the true goal.

3. **Achorya (honesty) :** Achorya means not to steal others' belongings (money or material), or use them without permission, or even a thought for one's own benefit in any way, or beyond the period permitted. This also includes breach of trust, misappropriation or misconduct. Its practice relieves a person from mental tensions, social evils and creates a harmonious atmosphere.

4. **Brahmacharya (sexual continence):** To adopt self-restraint is to lead the life of celibacy. It does not mean to completely abstain from sexual activities and not to lead a marital life at all. One must remain under limit, with one's own wife or husband, considering it as a duty for procreation and not for pleasure.

5. **Aparigraha (minimising desires) :** A yogic practitioner must keep his requirements to a minimum without a sense of hoarding. Collection of articles for future use reflects lack of faith in the Almighty, who looks after and cares for fulfilment of needs of all the living beings in the whole universe. Aparigraha makes one's life very simple, free from fear and frustrations, and one remains happy and satisfied with the belongings he has, with a sense of peace and in a state of equilibrium.

Niyama

It also contains five rules, as follows :-

1. **Shauch (purity) :** Besides cleanliness of the physical body, purity of mind from all anger, hatred, passion, lust, greed, pride etc. is shauch. Food should be satvik, that is simple, vegetarian, juicy, nourishing and not heavy. Atmosphere of the surroundings must be pollution free, that is free of insects or noise, and should be dry and clean. It helps the yoga practitioner to enter his own temple, to see one's own self in the mirror of one's own mind.

2. **Santosh (contentment) :** To develop a sense of contentment (satisfaction) is called santosh. Dissatisfaction and greed leads the mind to disturbance; hence one should always be satisfied with one's posessions, and concentrate on one's goal.

3. **Tapas (devotion to God) :** It involves self-purification, self-control, self-discipline and making efforts to achieve the ultimate union with the divine. Tapas involves body, speech and mind.

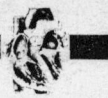

Brahmacharya and ahimsa become the parts of tapas. Tapas helps one to attain strength for body, mind and character.

4. **Swadhyaya (self-learning) :** Self-study or self-education is called swadhyaya. Education for the self by the self, without the need of any class-room or lecture hall, is called swadhyaya. The practitioner is a lecturer as well as a listener. By constant learning and reflection, one becomes noble at heart, developing a feeling of divinity in one's own self.

5. **Ishwar pranidhana (dedication) :** Full faith and surrender of self to God, with dedication of all desires, wishes and actions, is called pranidhana (samarpan). It implies worship of God, chanting His name, thinking of Him as the omnipresent entity. This requires extra strength, for which one has to take shelter of God with full dedication, reflecting : 'I am insignificant and the almighty will take care of me.' This method of bhakti will enable the practitioner to proceed in the right direction of knowledge and conduct. Name of God is like the sun : when our life-moon will be attracted to the sun, it will glow like a full moon.

Asanas

The daily practice of asanas is essential for keeping the body fit and pure as well as the mind in control. Maharshi Patanjali says, "स्थिरं सुखमासनम्", which means the asana is to sit in a posture that is comfortable and keeps the body straight and firm. To impart a state of effortless-ness to the body, to keep the body and mind away from overindulgence in worldly affairs and to provide necessary rest is the object of asana.

Regular practice of asanas results in the purification of veins and nerves and improvement in general health. The asanas are mainly of two types : (i) for meditation such as Padmasana, Siddhasana etc. and (ii) for physical health such as Bhujangasana, Pawan-muktasana etc. They tone up the entire body system and provide it strength and vigour.

The asanas are altogether different from gymnastic exercises or so-called western exercises. No additional infrastructure, facility or equipment is required to perform asanas as required in case of gymnastic exercises or other games. Asanas can be easily performed alone, anywhere and without any specific preparation. What is required is only a small sheet *(dari)* or a blanket, a clean and airy space and self-confidence.

Asanas besides securing a fine physique, keep the body free from disease and reduce fatigue. They smoothen the nervous system and lead to various useful physiological and biochemical changes in the body. These changes include loss of excessive body weight, decrease in respiratory rate, increase in vital capacity of lungs, expansion of chest, decrease in blood glucose and cholesterol levels, increase in blood protein and high-density lipid (HDL) levels, improvement in functions of endocrine glands and mental functions, that is mental quotient (M.Q.) and intelligence quotient (I.Q.). But their special importance lies in the quality that it trains and disciplines the mind. A perfect balance between physical and mental consciousness leads to perfect health.

As a matter of fact, health is not a commodity that can be purchased by spending money; it has to be achieved by sincere efforts, systematic hard work and practice. Asanas are the appropriate means for that. Asanas not only help a practioner to get free from physical and mental distractions, but also to achieve a complete equilibrium of body, mind and spirit.

Pranayama

Pranayama in short means 'yogic breathing', a systematic and disciplined breathing. Pranayama is related with 'prana' (the vital force), which means the life energy or life strength. The suffix 'ayam' means length, expansion, stretching or restraint. Pranayama thus means long and deep breathing with a control thereon. Pranayama activates Sushumna (spinal cord) and influences the entire nervous system, thereby developing the latent powers of the person, which can perform miracles.

Manu says, "दह्यन्ते ध्यायमानानां धातूनां हि यथा मलाः। तथेन्द्रियाणां दह्यन्ते दोषाः प्राणस्य निग्रहात्।।" That is, just as impurities of gold etc. are removed by the flame of fire, the senses throw out their impurities through pranayama.

Technique of pranayama : There are three components of every breath : (i) Puraka (inhalation), (ii) Rechaka (exhalation), and (iii) Kumbhaka (retention or holding of breath). Holding the breath after filling the lungs in Puraka stage is called Antarik Kumbhaka, and holding the breath outside in Rechaka stage is called Bahya Kumbhaka.

In pranayama there is a measured timing ratio for the three stages, and the ratio must be carefully observed. In yogic breathing Puraka consists of double muscular action. In the first part the thoracic cage expands to make room for the lungs to inflate. In the second part the dome-shaped diaphragm flattens out and descends, massaging beneficially the abdomial viscera. Hence one should breathe deeply and pour air into the lungs.

While performing pranayama if one sits comfortably with the back straight, the respiratory muscles become free to expand and are able to recoil easily. Holding of breath is a conscious act that checks the mechanism regulating our respiratory system automatically. During Kumbhaka, with the lungs full or empty, one achieves both physiological and psychological benefits through exchange of oxygen and carbon dioxide across the blood capillaries. In addition, it allows better mixing of fresh air with the residual air in the sacs of the lungs, resulting in better purification, more inflow of oxygen and greater intake of vital force.

Pratyahara (control over senses)

If a man is able to control one's senses, he may be free from several agonies. This is known as pratyahara. His purpose of life is to acquire the 'good' instead of 'pleasure'. But the common man goes for pleasure, losing the sacred element of precious life. Achievement of good and sacred is the ultimate goal of life. By practicing pratyahara, one feels joy and satisfaction, because he knows where to go and where to stop, what to accept and what to reject. He understands that, what appears poison (vish) today will become nectar (amirt) tomorrow.

By observing pratyahara, a person experiences the fullness of creation or the Creator. He remains in the state of equanimity, experiencing the fullness of the Universal Soul, and such a condition leads him to perfection.

Dharana (concentration)

Dharana is the elementary stage of meditation, i.e. concentration on a single point or total attention on what is to be done at a particular moment with the mind unmoved and unfurled. Dharna stimulates the inner awareness to integrate the ever-flowing intelligence and to release all tension. In fact, without concentration nothing can be achieved.

As a matter of fact, after yama, niyama and asanas, pranayama and pratyahara are practiced, one should be able to concentrate well and his mind should become a `willing servant'. But usually the mind is either a helpless slave or a tyrannical master. Our ancient yogis were very well aware of this problem and they wisely deviced a method to overcome it, which forms the basis of dharna. In the process of dharna one should focus one's full attention on a specific image or object determinedly, shutting out everything else.

In the first instance when one begins to concentrate on some object of one's choice, immediately there is a pre-conception of daily routine crowding the mental faculty. The way to tackle these thoughts is to simply watch them as a silent spectator, without identifying with them. The thoughts of day-dreaming, wool-gathering etc. would vanish away. It will be really surprising how quickly this mechanical exercise enables the person to discipline his mind to focus on something specifically important, according to his will.

Those who want to achieve success in dharna should regulate their diet, thinking, speech and actions first, and then practice dharna (concentration) with perfect dedication daily. The regularity and punctuality will be additional factors in achieving the goal.

Dhyana (meditation)

Meditation is the practice of constant observation of mind, focusing it on a single point. Focusing the sun-rays with a mangnifying glass makes them hot enough, as is obvious in solar-power appliances. By focusing the scattered rays of thought they work collectively and make the mind powerful. By regular and continuous practice of meditation, one can develop will power and strengthen it.

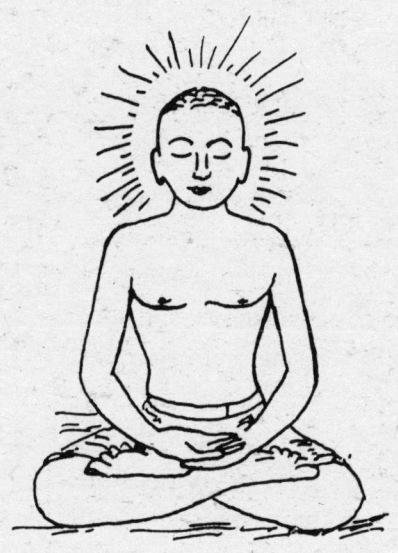

Fig. 10.1 A state of meditation

In *Vivek Chudamani* it has been stated that dhyana purifies the mind from Rajas and Tamas gunas and enlightens the mind with Satva guna, similar to an alkali that purifies gold and makes it bright and sparkling. One's thinking thus becomes clearer and more concentrated. Through meditation one gains the sense of perspective to accept the hard facts and gauge the good and bad. Sense of jealousy or ego, resentment or hatred, weakness or defeat, insecurity or fear, which are the root causes of physical and psychosomatic disorders, vanish away.

However, in meditation one must not hurry and be anxious for early results. As a beautiful tree grows gradually, meditation gives results slowly, but the blossom of meditation is an inexpressible event that permeates the entire being.

Samadhi

Samadhi is the climax of dhyana (super consciousness and perfect calm). When dhyana matures, subject and object become one. This helps the seeker to unfold the world of knowledge and wisdom, where he loses all consciousness of body, breathing, mind, intelligence and ego. He reaches the superconscious state, where his wisdom and purity shine forth.

10.5 Preksha Yoga (Seven steps)

In this age of technology, industrialisation and overurbanisation, people are constantly subjected to tremendous stress and tension. These, in turn, produce psychosomatic diseases like hypertension, insomnia and various types of heart ailments. In desperation, people take tranquilisers, drinks, various drugs or smoke, which gives temporary apparent relief, but creates more serious problems. The remedy does not lie in drugs or fantasy, but in the development of the inherent power. Preksha meditation (P.M.)

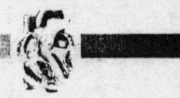

is an easy technique to overcome these problems.

We should realise that our existence is functioning in duality, i.e. there is a spiritual self within the physical body. Life's processes for man lie almost wholly within himself and are amenable to control. The control has to be exercised by the power of spiritual self, and that inherent potency can be developed by knowing how to live properly, which includes eating, drinking, breathing as well as thinking properly.

What is preksha meditation?

Preksha meditation is a technique of perceptive meditation for attitudinal change, behavioural modification and integrated development of personality. It is based on the wisdom of ancient philosophy and has been formulated in terms of modern scientific concepts.

The word *'preksha'* is a sanskrit word, which means to *'perceive carefully and profoundly'*.

Here, *'seeing'* does not mean external vision, but careful concentration on subtle consciousness by mental insight. In other words, in this system of meditation one's mind is fully concentrated in the perception of subtle internal and innate phenomenon of consciousness.

The term *'dhyana'* (meditation) is usually defined as the concentration of thinking on a particular subject for a length of time. Now, the mind is the instrument of *'thinking'* as well as *'perception'*. Therefore, when linked with *'preksha'*, meditation becomes concentration of perception and not of thought.

Aims and objectives of preksha meditation

The main purpose of the practice of preksha meditation is to purify the mental states. Mind is constantly choked by contaminating urges, emotions and passions. This hampers the flow of wisdom. The hurdles of uncleanliness must first be removed. When the mind is purged of all contaminations, peace of mind automatically surfaces. Balance of mind, equanimity and the state of well-being are also established.

Thus preksha meditation is a technique for controlling one's irrational instincts of anger, aggressiveness, cruelty, vindictiveness and fear. It is a tool for awakening and developing one's conscious reasoning and thereby modifying one's attitude and behaviour. As the irrational instincts and impulses emanate from the endocrines, and not the brain, a pious resolution or mere intellectual knowledge is not potent enough to destroy an evil. Perceptive meditation strengthens the power of rational thinking and weakens the irrational impulses and primal drives. As a by-product, one gains physical health and cures serious illnesses without the use of injurious drugs. The regular practice of preksha meditation is ultimately responsible for homoestasis in the body.

The ultimate aim of preksha meditation is purity and equanimity—freedom from contamination of passions. To obtain the state of well-being and peacefulness is not our ultimate goal, although it will inevitably ensue. We have to transcend both these mental states to reach our ultimate purpose, viz. total purity of mind and goodness.

Seven steps of preksha meditation

1. **Kayotsarga (total relaxation with self-awareness) :** To concentrate the mind on each and every part of the body, one by one, starting from the toe up-to the head, and to achieve relaxation of each part through auto-suggestion is called **kayotsarga.**

2. **Antaryatra (internal trip through spinal cord and brain) :** In the second step, the conscious mind is allowed to travel inside the spinal cord, upwards from its lower end up to the brain and again downwards up to the lower end of spinal cord.

3. **Shwas preksha (perception of breathing) :** It involves concentration of one's mind on breathing, i.e. each inhalation and exhalation, making it deep, slow, calm and rhythmic. Such a complete breathing is achieved through diaphragmatic breathing, i.e. allowing the abdominal muscles to contract and expand respectively during each exhalation and inhalation, and thus allowing to raise and lower the diaphragm and facilitate the lungs to use their maximum vital capacity.

4. **Sharir preksha (perception of body):** It requires concentration of one's mind on the subtle intrinsic phenomenon occurring in each and every part of the body, one by one. One perceives various chemical, mechanical and electro-magnetic processes taking place within each and every cell of the body. The process is centripetal, i.e. from outside to inside. The successive stages of the exercise would be perception and awareness of the superficial sensation of skin, such as contact with clothes, warmth, itching, perspiration, sensations of muscular movements, deeper sensations in the internal organs and subtle vibrations of electrical impulses in the nervous system.

5. **Chaitanya kendra preksha (perception of psychic centres) :** It means concentration of mind on certain 'psychic centres'. There are some points in our body where psychic energy is more concentrated. These are called psychic centres. Perception of psychic centres means 'focusing of full attention on these centres and perceiving them with deep concentration'. These centres are associated with our endocrine glands. The endocrines exert profound influence on the mental state and behaviour of an individual. These psychic centres are the fields of consciousness, influencing the endocrine and the nervous systems of our body.

6. **Leshya dhyana (perception of psychic colours) :** In the next step one practices colour meditation, which is called '*Leshya dhyana*'. It is the perception of psychic

colours. In this practice we perceive a specific colour on a specific psychic centre. Table 10.1 shows the psychic centres and colours to be visualized and what is to be experienced by intense willing.

7. **Therapeutic thinking through auto-suggestion and contemplation :** The system of preksha meditation bifurcates into : (a) concentration of perception, and (b) concentration of thought, i.e. 'Preksha' and `Anupreksha'. In the former, perception is primarily used for concentration whereas in the latter the conscious mind is encouraged to concentrate on a thinking process, i.e. contemplation. Auto-suggestions during meditation increase the inner strength of an individual to choose the right type of food and enjoy it and feel empowered to give up eating his most favourite dishes. He can let go of his favourite dairy products, rich chocolate or ice-cream without feeling the sense of deprivation and experience the fact that he can now do without it. Both the techniques are competent to develop the practitioner's conscious reasoning and modify one's attitude and behaviour. Auto-suggestion practiced during Anupreksha brings about a desired change in physical, mental or emotional conditions. It is a valuable exercise for curing disorders and diseases, and also for developing positive attitudes.

Table 10.1 Psychic centres in the body and colours to be visualized during leshya dhyana

	Psychic centre	Colour to be visualized	Intense willing and experience
I.	Centre of bliss (Anand Kendra) Anahata Chakra	Emerald green	Freedom from psychological faults and negative attitudes
II.	Centre of purity (Vishuddhi Kendra) Vishuddhi Chakra	Peacock-neck blue	Self-control of urges and impulses (specially the sexual distortions)
III.	Centre of intuition (Darshan Kendra) : Agya Chakra	Rising-sun red	Awakening of intuition and bliss, strong will power
IV.	Centre of wisdom (Gyan Kendra) Sahasrara Chakra	Golden yellow	Acuity of perception, clarity of thought, improvement in memory power
V.	Centre of enlightenment (Jyoti Kendra) Agya Chakra	Full-moon white	Tranquility, peace, subsidence of agitation, excitation, anger, etc.

Visualization is an imaginative process of forming pictures in the mind's eye. When we visualize in a non-meditative mood, i.e. when our mind is full of other thoughts, visualizaiton is not effective because it is unfocused and passive. However, during meditation, visualization becomes active and focused. It is like the sunrays converging through a magnifying glass and burning the paper. Visualzation during meditation brings about the desired effects. A CHD patient may visualize as to how their coronary circulation and function of tthe heart may improve and how he feels energetic in his daily routine. The beauty of this visualization is that, though there may be no anatomical or physiological relevance to his imagination, it still impoves the clinical condition of the patient. Dr Dean Ornish has also noted it to be useful to his patients.

10.6 Benefits of Preksha Yoga

1. Mental happiness and experience of religiosity.
2. Physical benfits like radical change in body chemistry.
3. Psychic benefits like change of habit or change of heart.
4. Benefits in perception of breathing: Greater alertness and concentration, improvement in operational efficiency, energy generation, retardation of ageing.
5. Benefits of perception of body : Even-ness of the vitality, rejuvenation of the body, enhancement of immunity, increased vigilance, transmutation of personality, higher level of consciousness, freedom from psychological distortions.
6. Benefits of perception of psychic centres : Stimulation of the centre of joy, purification of character, strengthening of will power, and control as well as transmutation of anger, hatred, selfishness, jealousy, fear etc.
7. Benefits of perception of psychic colours: Virtuous and decent behaviour, delighted living, commencement of transmutation, ineffable and innate happiness, cessation of mental weakness, reinforcement of brain and nervous system, and freedom from anguish and infatuation.
8. Benefit of contemplation and auto suggestion : Freedom from sickness and negative attitudes, attainment of bliss and development of positive attitude.
9. All the above benefits help the heart work more efficiently.

10.7 Benefits of Kayotsarga

First stage : In the first stage of relaxation, one learns to keep still and stop all voluntary movements. The turmoil due to restlessness vanishes and an acute sense of relaxation and relief from tension is experienced. There is progressive improvement in treatment of psychosomatic diseases such as hypertension. Physically it is more restful than sleep and it is the direct antidote to these diseases.

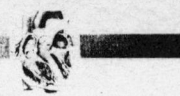

Second stage : In the second stage of relaxation, some further benefits occur.

1. There is a soothing effect on the nervous system.
2. Change in the electrical activity of the nervous system (soothing alpha waves may be produced at will).
3. Rate of metabolism slows down and the need for oxygen is greatly reduced.
4. Control is established on the in - voluntary or smooth internal muscles. The level of excitation of these muscles is reduced and they are less tense.
5. Operational efficiency increases.
6. There is an increase in the capacity for bearing environmental changes such as heat and cold.
7. Sharpens the intellect.
8. Concentration is easily achieved.

Third stage : In the third stage, self-awareness increases and the physical body remains in the background. The subtle body is clearly identified and sometimes it can be separated from the gross body. Perception is more acute and is considerably more obvious than the proverbial five senses.

Fourth stage : In the fourth and final stage, the separateness of the body and spiritual self is complete. Self-awareness becomes constant without any hindrance.

Achievements from Kayotsarga

Relief from tension : The most obvious and measurable benefit from relaxation is elimination of tension. Any- body who practices regular kayotsarga (relaxation) will get rid of his tension in a short time and will achieve the stage of relaxation (calm and unperturbed state in any situation). It not only relieves you from tension but also revitalise the body. Heaviness and congestion fade away and the practitioner enjoys a feeling of well-being and lightness. More significant is the relief from mental load and heaviness. Regular practitioner achieves a superior personality and never suffers form mental disorders.

Freedom from turmoil : Normally our body is constantly agitated in turmoil. Electric impulses keep the muscles magnetised and contracted. There is no rest. Relaxation starts when there is suspension of all movements of the skeletal muscles.

These vital activities of the body are the province of autonomous nervous system and are not generally under voluntary control. But as relaxation progresses, these activities also calm down. Breathing, heart beat and the circulation of blood slow down. Rate of energy metabolism is reduced and the need for oxygen is greatly cut down. As the exercise continues, the muscles begin to relax and drain out the tension, turmoil gets reduced and in due course it completely vanishes. All the needs and necessities of the organism are reduced to a minimum and an unprecedented peacefulness prevails in the absence of turmoil.

Revitalisation of the organism : On the physical level, benefits of relaxation are obvious and measurable. The sensory nerves are always loaded with the continuous task of collecting and despatching information. Motor nerves are similarly engaged in transmitting messages from the brain to the muscles, glands and other tissues, and producing action. The work is tiring and there is no respite. Relaxation provides the much-needed rest to the nerves and neurons. They become free from the load of their onerous duties. This rest gives them a chance of recuperating. The flow of vital energy saved from being wasted in producing tension now revitalises and rejuvenates every tissue and cell. There is no wander; therefore relaxation can relieve fatigue more effectively in a few minutes than in hours of indifferent sleep. It will also be clear from the above that sleep, during exercise of relaxation, is considered a distraction. However, relaxation may be performed just before retiring for the night to get a more restful sleep.

Those who face the risk of heart diseases because of blood pressure can strengthen their resistance by practising relaxation. In an experimental study it was concluded that when 100 electronic factory workers, in risk of developing heart diseases because of their high blood pressure, cholesterol level or smoking habits, were given an hour's relaxation session, once a week for 8 weeks, their B.P. decreased significantly. Three years later these workers had maintained lower blood pressure and had suffered fewer incidences of heart disease than that of a controlled group of patients who had received conventional treatment.

Self-awareness : When the turmoil of the body ceases and one achieves total absence of motion, there is an acute state of self-awareness. The body is forgotten and the **spiritual self** reveals its separate existence. This is neither imagination nor auto-suggestion but a real experience. The experience is characterised by an actual feeling of floating outside one's body. This is self-awareness, leading to self-realisation.

Development of aura : Every object living or non-living is surrounded by its aura, the envelope of its electro-magnetic radiation. This is normally invisible to the naked eyes. The aura of a living being is interaction of material and psychic radiation. In the profound state of relaxation, the aura becomes perceptable. This perception is partly sensory and partly extra-sensory. When the motionless state is perfect, the ingress from external environment is minimal. In this state, the consciousness transcends the physical body and one becomes aware of the activities of the subtle inner body. The awareness of the subtle body affects attitudinal changes.

Yogic Cure to Avoid Heart Surgery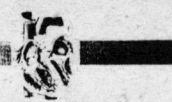

Development of wisdom : Wisdom constitutes discernment of material from non-material, body from soul, and the physical self from the spiritual self. Body is material, self is non-material. Body is perishable, self is eternal. The separation is real when wisdom develops. It is a great achievement and the benefit arises from kayotsarga.

Wisdom is different from intelligence in that the latter is replete with likes and dislikes : this is pleasant and that is unpleasant. Wisdom transcends the duality of like and dislike, attachment and detachment. Equanimity and tranquility take the place of like and dislike. The benefit derived from relaxation is substitution of intelligence by wisdom. As wisdom matures, intelligence takes a back seat and transcendence of gain-loss, pleasure-pain, criticism-adulation, life-death, and such other dualities is effortless. The dualities are replaced by a single entity instead, i.e. equanimity and bliss.

CHAPTER 11

Yogic Management of Coronary Heart Disease in India and Abroad

Contents

11.1	Dean Ornish's concept of CHD reversal through yoga	109
11.2	Treatment of CHD through yoga in India	110

Yogic Management of Coronary Heart Disease in India and Abroad

11.1 Dean Ornish's Concept of CHD Reversal

Dr Dean Ornish from the USA formulated a plan of life-style to combat heart diseases, which produced remarkable results in the reversal of CHD. He treated his patients without any surgical process. He adopted the following four strategies:

1. **Stress management :** He started to educate his patients to live a stress-free life comprising yoga, meditation, imagery and pranayama (breathing exercise) all together for an hour a day, for 60 days.

2. **Aerobic exercises :** Light aerobic exercises, which were very convenient, for about half an hour a day for 60 days.

3. **Non-smoking :** He advised the patients to stop smoking completely.

4. **Pure vegetarian diet :** He asked his patients to take pure vegetarian food with low fat content.

Though this strategy appears very simple, it gave tremendous success. It proves that `**the greatest truths are the simplest ones**'.

Dr Dean Ornish made all the relevant data of his results available in the latest medical gadget, `Pet Scan', to prove his reversal theory. This scientific report was again published in 1995 in the *Journal of Amercian Medical Association.* The whole medical scientific world had to give him at least an attentive listening. The theory became much more popular and today Dr Dean Ornish's name is famous throughout the world for reversal of heart disease without surgical assistance. He offers his reversal programmes in eight major hospitals in the USA including Harward Medical School, Boston and Beth Israel Hospital, New York city.

Yogic Cure to Avoid Heart Surgery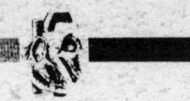

11.2 Treatment of C.H.D. through Yoga in India

Here, in India, some doctors are also running, a Heart Disease Reversal Programme on the pattern of the one started by Dr Dean Ornish. One, Dr Chhajer, is conducting heart disease-reversal programme camp for the last few years in New Delhi and other metropolitan cities of India. This 5-day residential programme is known as SAAOL Heart Programme. It includes the following key components:

1. Yogic exercises
2. Asanas and pranayama
3. Preksha dhyana
4. Stress management
5. Dietary management

Both Dr Dean Ornish and Dr chhajer had conclusively proved that reversal without surgery is actually possible. But the success depends only on the right combination of theory and practice, depending on the environment where the patient belongs. It was revealed that 90% of the patients who had attended such non-invasive programmes at any yoga training centre had never had a heart attack, the most dreaded or feared complication of coronary heart disease.

Swami Dharma Nand Ji, Director, Adhyatm Sadhna Kendra, Chhatarpur Road, Mehrauli, New Delhi also organises one week yoga camps every fortnight for treatment of Coronary Heart Disease through yoga at his Ashram. The cases where bypass surgery is advised, but can not be done for many a reason, are also entertained there. Many a people are being benefited by his programe. The results are very encouraging.

Dr. S.C. Manchanda Cardiologist, All India Institute of Medical Sciences, New Delhi alongwith his team also associates him.

The development in medical technology or a very big hospital could take care of much of the sufferings of the society, but how many of us can afford the technology like that, especially with our socioeconomic set-up? It is astonishing to discover that such superstructures providing expensive surgery or angioplasty cater to even less then 2% of our population of cardiac patients in India. Thus such CHD-reversal programmes, as being conducted by Dean Ornish, SAAOL and Swami Dharma Nand Ji, should be promoted throughout India.

Section 5

Dietary Management

CHAPTER 12

Dietary Management

Contents

12.1	Role of diet in managing CHD	115
12.2	Nutrients	116
12.3	CHD reversal diet	117
12.4	Anti-oxidants of food	117
12.5	An ideal food chart for CHD patients	118
	➢ Breakfast, lunch, evening tea, dinner	
12.6	How to prepare zero-oil food	119
12.7	Food items	121
	➢ Restricted, moderately restricted, freely consumable	

Dietary Management

12.1 Role of Diet in Managing CHD

Diet plays a very important role in the formation of blockage in the coronary arteries. The type of food we eat, the quantity of food we consume, of course has a direct relationship with our daily calorie requirement. Diet also has a bifactorial relationship with coronary heart disease. First, it is related in terms of calories (energy) and second in terms of fat intake.

This is quite simple to understand, if we think for a moment about total energy intake in terms of calories, comparing the calories (energy) we spend every day. Suppose the total amount of calories spent in a day is 1600, then we eat much more than our daily requirment (Table 12.1). This is a common tendency of everyone. We never consume less than the daily required calories to perfom routine duties. Since we are in the habit of consuming excess food every time (eating something or the other all the time), the extra intake is stored in the form of fat, which also gets deposited not only in the body but also in the inner lining of the blood vessels. Over a long period of time, cholesterol deposition in blood vessels gradually increases, giving rise to severe obstruction to blood flow through these vessels, which ultimately results in coronary artery disease.

Food rich in fats such as egg yolk, mutton, fish, ghee, butter, milk, nuts and dry fruits are responsible for the elevation in blood-cholesterol level (Table 12.2). It is thus important to pay particular attention to the `diet' in the management of coronary artery disease. If this aspect is neglected, the blockages in blood vessels of the heart will continue to increase in size in spite of all efforts to treat the disease medically or surgically.

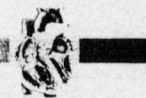

Table 12.1 Physical activities and approximate calorie consumption

Activity	Energy expenditure (calories/minute)
Sleeping	0.8
Reading	1.4
Eating	1.8
Discussing	1.8
Sitting/writing	2.0
Driving a car	2.1
Standing	2.2
Walking (casual)	4-5
Walking (brisk)	6-8
Jogging	7-9
Playing football	7-10
Running	10-12

12.2 Nutrients

Man needs a wide range of nutrients to perfom various functions in the body and to lead a healthy life. The nutrients include carbohydrates, proteins, fats, vitamins and minerals. Calories of the basic nutrients are given here.

Diet	Calories
Carbohydrates	4 cal. per gram
Proteins	4 cal. per gram
Fats	9 cal. per gram

Vitamins and minerals do not yield energy, but they play a very important and significant role in regulating the metabolic activities in the body. Hence the diet must be well balanced, containing all the nutrients in a proper proportion.

Table 12.2 Cholesterol contents in food

Food	Approximate contents
Meat, chicken, fish	100 mg/100 gm
Liver, kidney	300 mg/100 gm
Brain	200 mg/100 gm
Egg	250 mg/one
Egg (white)	0 mg/one
Milk	40 mg/glass
Ice-cream	50 mg/small cup
Butter/ghee	35 mg/tablespoon
Fish oil	500 mg/tablespoon
Vegetable oil	0 mg/100 gm (but full of triglycerides)
Nuts, oilseeds	0 mg/100 gm (but full of triglycerides)

Dietary Management

Typical diet per day contains :

40 to 50% fat (mostly saturated).

25 to 35% carbohydrate.

25% proteins.

400-500 milligrams cholesterol.

An ideal diet per day for CHD patients:

10% fat (invisible form)

70 to 75% carbohydrate

15 to 20% proteins

5 milligrams cholesterol

12.3 CHD Reversal Diet

Diet forms an important part of yogic lifestyle intervention programme. The subjects (CHD patients) should take a diet low in fat (mostly poly or unsatured, providing 15% calories), low in cholesterol (less than 50 mg daily) and high in carbohydrate (mostly complex, providing 65% calories). They should take high soluble fibre dite consisting of vegetables and fruits, oat bran, soyabean, gram and other beans. They may also take 15 gm isabgol husk daily.

In addition, the diet should be rich in anti-oxidants.

12.4 Anti-oxidants of Food

Free radicals are the by-product of oxidation. When oxygen is used by the body, it burns food to produce energy. It also burns germs and toxic substances such as ozone and carbon monoxide. In the process, free radicals are produced. These radicals damage the cell membrane, disturb chromosomes and genetic material and destroy valuable enzymes, causing a chain reaction of damage throughout the body. Thus free radicals are the major cause of at least 50% diseases such as coronary heart disease, lung disease, certain cancers, cataract, rheumatoid arthritis and Parkinson's disease.

Vitamin A is needed for growth and for keeping the body tissues healthy. One of its most important roles is to reinforce the protective envelope or membrane that surrounds all our cells. It also protects the mucous membrane. It is fat soluble.

Beta carotene is one of the most powerful anti-oxidants that prevents plants from burning up in the ultraviolet rays of the sun—nature's perfect antidote. Fruits and vegetables that contain beta-carotene are melons, apricots, peaches, mangoes, carrots, parsley (raw), sweet potato, spinach, watercress (raw), spring greens, tomatoes, asparagus and broccoli (cabbage).

Vitamin C (ascorbic acid) possesses many extraordinary properties. without which we are liable to many infections and can even die of scurvy. Chemically speaking, vitamin C is one of the simplest vitamins. It helps in the growth and repair of the body tissues and gums, blood vessels, bones and teeth. It is involved in the functioning of the immune system and helps the body to fight off bacteria and viral infections.

Vitamin E is a fighter free radical, because it protects every cell in the body. It is the virility vitamin, because it plays an important role in human fertility. It improves the immune system by strengthening the white blood cells and helps in the prevention of heart disease.

12.5 An Ideal Food Chart for CHD Patients

Breakfast

(25% of the total K cal. for the day)

1. Prefer brown bread; also chapaties, preferably with choker and G.L.V.
2. Salad in any form must be taken daily.
3. Prefer ayurvedic herbal tea to regular tea.
4. Fruits as chaat and whole fruit.
5. Skimmed or toned milk (200 to 250 ml a day).

Lunch

(35% of the total K cal. for the day)

1. First course should be salad. Salad should contain, lemon, vinegar, tomato, amla, onion and chutney.
2. For chapaties, perfer wheat flour mixed with chana dal flour or soya flour and G.L.V.
3. Spices (masalas) according to the individuals's taste.
4. Lay stress on alteration and combination of various pulses.

Evening tea

(15% of the total K cal. for the day)

1. Prefer herbal tea to normal tea.
2. Consume low-calorie snack items like murmura, popcorn, khil, rice flakes, poha, upma, fruit chats, sprouts (gram or greengram), steamed items like dhokla or idli, Marie biscuits etc.

Dinner

(25% of the total K cal. for the day)

1. Salad should be the first course.
2. Dinner should always be taken 2 hours before bed time.
3. It should be the lightest of all meals.
4. Try to include soups during dinner.
5. For 100% dinner, the stomach is to be filled with :

    40% food (chapaties etc.)

    20% salad

    20% water

    20 % empty.

Substitue conventional sweet dishes with fruits, washed amla murabba and washed petha mithai.

Dietary Management

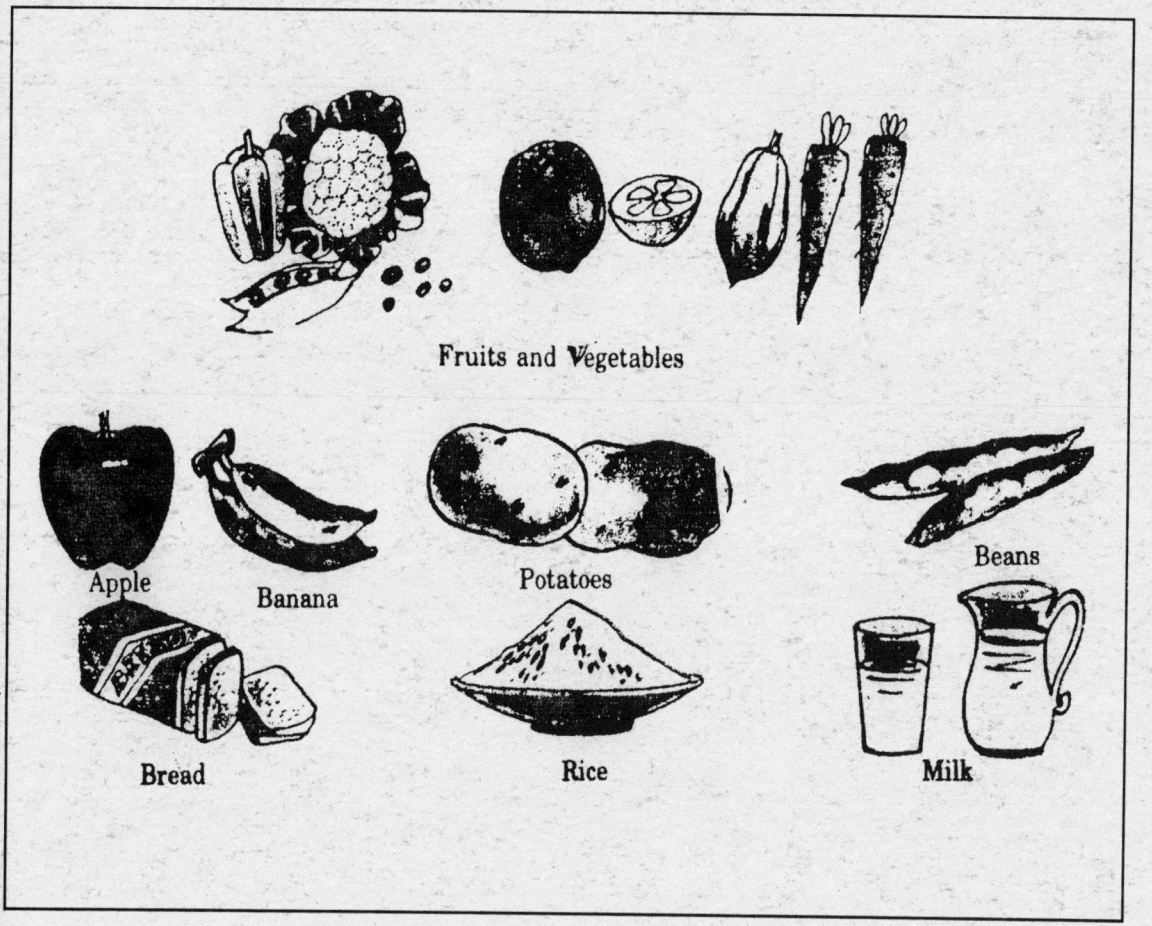

Fig. 12.1 Useful food items

12.6 How to Prepare Zero-oil Food

The National Institute of Nutrition (NIN), Hyderabad recommends that minimum 10% of calories required in our body should come from fat, consisting of vegetable oils, rich essential fatty acids (EFA). This will help lower the blood-cholesterol level. Hydrogenated fats and vegetable fats with low EFA content should be avoided. To aviod any futher risk to CHD patients, the doctors and experts recommend least oil consumption or no oil. Water therefore should be used for cooking food, instead of oil; hence it is called zero-oil food. The addition of raw oil in our food is not required at all. To prepare zero-oil food, two recipes are being given here under.

Yogic Cure to Avoid Heart Surgery

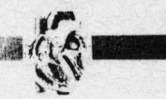

1. Rajma masala

Ingredients

Rajma (boiled)	- 1 cup
Onion (chopped)	- 1/4 cup
Tomato sauce	- 1/4 cup
Garlic paste	- 1/2 cup
Cumin powder	- 1 tsf
Coriander powder	- 1 tsf
Salt and pepper	- To taste
Chilli powder	- 1/2 tsf

Method

1. In a pan saute onion and garlic paste. Put a little water and simmer till the liquid evaporates.
2. Stir in boiled rajma, tomato sauce, cumin powder, coriander powder, chilli powder, salt and pepper.
3. Simmer for 15-20 minutes stirring occasionally till done.
4. This can be used as such or as a filling in kadhi rolls.

Nutritive value (approx.) :

(1 medium katori)

Energy	- 119 calories
Carbohydrates	- 21.86 gm
Protein	- 7.26 gm
Fat	- 0.43 gm

2. Vegetable upma

Ingredients

Semolina	- 1 cup
Peas (steamed)	- 1/4 cup
Carrot (grated)	- 1/4 cup
Onion (chopped)	- 1/4 cup
Mustard seeds	- 1/4 cup
Curry leaves	- 4-5 leaves
Chana dal	- 1/2 tsp
Urad dal	- 1/2 tsp
Salt	- To taste
Coriander leaves	- 2 tsp
Red chilli powder	- 1/4 tsp

Method

1. Dry roast the semolina lightly and keep aside.
2. Now roast mustard seeds, curry leaves, chana dal, urad dal and onion one by one.
3. To the roasted masala, add salt, steamed peas, grated carrot and roasted semolina.
4. Now add water and cook till done.
5. Serve with coriander and mint chutney.

Nutritive value (approx.) :

(1 quarter-plate)

Energy	- 155 calories
Carbohydrates	- 32.44 gm
Protein	- 5.40 gm
Fat	- 0.37 gm

Dietary Management

12.7 Food Items

Restricted

1. Milk (full cream) and milk products
2. Skimmed milk (bina vasa ka doodh) beyond 200 ml per day
3. Cheese and butter
4. Butter milk (lassi of skimmed milk) beyond 200 ml per day
5. All kinds of non-vegetarian items
6. Nuts and dry fruits
7. Sweets (mithai)
8. Oil (all types of oils)
9. Cold drinks (sheetal pay)

Moderately restricted

1. Brown bread and white bread (double roti)
2. Rice (chawal)
3. Vermicelli (sewai)
4. Pearl millet (bajra)
5. Sorghum (jowar)
6. Maize (makka)
7. Peas dry (matar sukha)
8. Potato, sweet potato (shakarkandi) arvi
9. Jaggery (gur)
10. Cane sugar (chini)
11. Banana ripe (kela)
12. Mango.

Freely consumable

Cereals

1. Rice puffed (murmura)
2. Rice, flakes (chirwa)

Pulses

3. Bengal gram whole (chana)
4. Bengal gram dal (chana ki dal)
5. Bengal gram, roasted (bhuna chana)
6. Black gram, dal (urad dal)
7. Cowpea (lobia)
8. Greengram, whole (moong)
9. Greengram dal (moong ki dal)
10. Horsegram, whole (kulthi)
11. Lentil (masoor)
12. Moth beans (moth)
13. Green peas (matar)
14. Rajmah (rajmah)
15. Red gram, (arhar dal)
16. soybean (bhatmas)

Leafy vegetables

17. Bathua leaves (bathua saag)
18. Spinach (palak)
19. Radish leaves (mooli ka saag)
20. Cabbage (patta gobhi)
21. Amaranth (cholai saag)

Yogic Cure to Avoid Heart Surgery

22. Carrot leaves (gajar saag)
23. Colocasia leaves (arvi ka saag)
24. Drumstick (saijan)
25. Fenugreek (methi saag)
26. Lettuce (salad leaves)
27. Mint (pudina)
28. Mustard leaves (sarson ka saag)

Roots and Tubers

29. Yam, ordinary (jamikand)
30. Carrot (gajar)
31. Onion (pyaj)
32. White radish (safed mooli)
33. Garlic
34. Ginger

Other vegetables

35. Beans (sem)
36. Brinjal (baingan)
37. Cucumber (khira)
38. French beans (bakla)
39. Lotus stem dry, (kamal kakari)
40. Parwar (parmal)
41. Pumpkin (kaddu)
42. Lady's finger (bhindi)
43. Round gourd (tinda)
44. Tomato (tamatar)
45. Bottle gourd (ghia)
46. Long gourd (torai)
47. Capsicum (shimla mirch)
48. Cucumber (kakri)
49. Mushrooms

Fruits

50. Apple (seb)
51. Guava (amrood)
52. Lemon (nimbu)
53. Orange (mousami)
54. Orange (santara)
55. Water melon (tarbooj)
56. Papaya ripe (papita)
57. Pineapple (anannas)
58. Tomato, ripe
59. Muskmelon (kharbooza)
60. Jambu fruit (jamun)
61. Raw mango
62. Plum (aloo bukhara)
63. Amla
64. Peach (nashpati).

Section 6

An Innovative Yogic Life-style Intervention Programme for CHD Management

CHAPTER 13

Innovative Yogic Life-style Intervention Programme for CHD Management

Contents

13.1	Introduction	127
13.2	Components of the programme	127
➢	Health-rejuvenating yogic exercises:	128
	(head and mind, eyes, neck, ears, face, shoulders, chest and lungs, waist, thighs and hips, feet, knees, ankles, toes and heels), kayotsarga	
➢	Yogic asanas	136
	(Tadasana, Padahastasana, Vajrasana, Sashankasana, Ardhchandrasana, Ardhamatsyendrasana, Uttanpadasana, Merudandasana, Bhujangasana, Shalabhasana, Pawanmuktasana)	
➢	General conditions for performing asanas	
➢	Benefits of asnas	
➢	Precautions for asanas	
➢	Pranayama (breathing exercise):	143
	abdominal breathing, anulom - vilom pramayama, om dhwani and laughter	
➢	Benefits of pranayama	
➢	Precautions for pranayama	
➢	Mudras:	146
	(apan mudra, vyan mudra)	
➢	Kayotsarga (total relaxation with self-awareness)	147
➢	Preksha Meditation	148
	(special meditation for CHD patients)	

Innovative Yogic Life-style Intervention Programme

13.1 Introduction

Yoga has been used as a successful therapy during the recent few decades. The researchers have proved that yoga has surpassed the medical science of chemicals and surgical knives. Yoga reduces the high blood pressure, high blood-cholesterol level and body weight without any side-effects, unlike other drugs. Yogic practices improve the physical fitness and working efficiency besides inducing mental happiness.

The latest research studies have shown that modification in life-style and food habits, yogic exercise and asanas, yogic relaxation and training in stress management not only reduce the risk of coronary heart disease but also reverse the disease itself.

The great philosopher Hippocrates says:

"All parts of the body which have a function, if used in moderation and exercised in which each is accustomed, become thereby healthy, well developed and age more slowly; but if misused and/or left idle, they become liable to disease, defective in growth and age quickly."

13.2 Components of the Programme

The proposed yogic life-style intervention programme consists of the following steps for the treatment of coronary heart disease :

1. Health-rejuvenating yogic exercises
2. Yogic asanas
3. Pranayama
4. Mudras
5. Kayotsarga
6. Special preksha meditation for CHD patients
7. Stress management (including positive thinking and reflection of moral values)
8. Diet management.

The detailed and step-by-step techniques of above mentioned compoments are being described here.

Yogic Cure to Avoid Heart Surgery

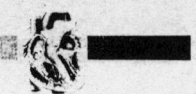

Health Rejuvenating Yogic Exercises

- **For head and mind (Fig. 13.1)**

Position : Stand erect, feet together, arms hanging down, and touching the thighs.

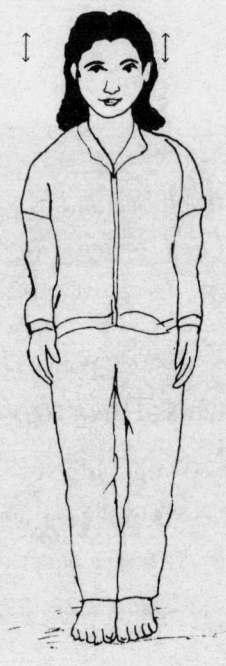

Fig. 13.1 Exercise for head and mind

Movements :

1. Concentrate upon forehead with eyeballs upward. Feel that brain cells are becoming active and full of life.
2. Now contract the muscles of fore-head and then relax.
3. Repeat contraction and relaxation 5 to 10 times.

- **For eyes (Fig. 13.2 a, b, c)**

Position : Stand erect and keep the neck stationary.

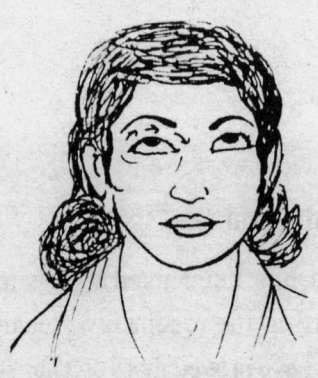

Fig. 13.2 a Exercise for eyes

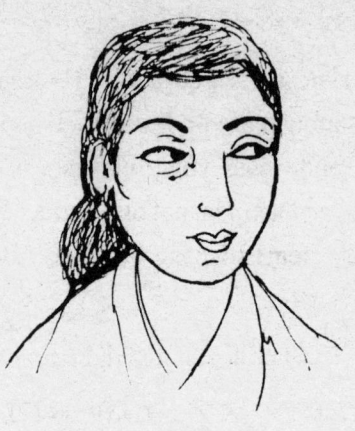

Fig. 13.2 b Exercise for eyes

Innovative Yogic Life-style Intervention Programme

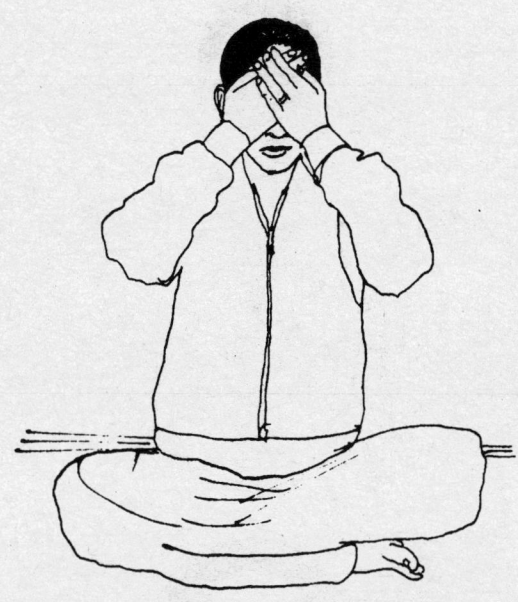

Fig. 13.2 c Exereice for eyes

- **For neck (Fig. 13.3 a, b, c)**

Position : Stand at ease and erect.

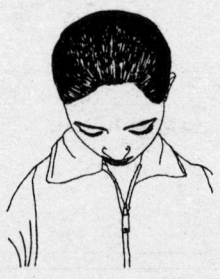

Fig. 13.3a Exercise for neck

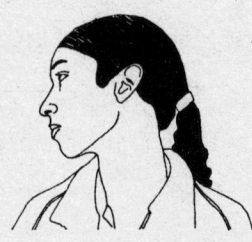

Fig. 13.3b Exercise for neck

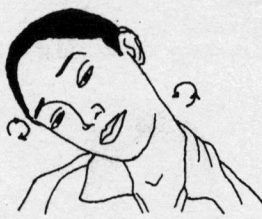

Fig. 13.3c Exercise for neck

Movements :

1. While inhaling, move your eyeballs upwards, towards the sky, and then while exhaling look at the feet alternately (Fig. 13.2 a).

2. Then look towards your right and left sides. Rotate your eyeballs only. Try to cover maximum range(Fig. 13.2 b).

3. Rotate your eyeballs in a circle clockwise, and anti-clockwise 5 times each.

4. Rub your palms to warm them, put on the eyes, making a dark cavity over the eyes, and then blink a few times (Fig. 13.2 c).

Movements :

1. Rub the palms together 10 times and then rub the front and back sides of the neck 5 times.

Yogic Cure to Avoid Heart Surgery

2. Inhale and bend your neck backwards to look at the sky. Then exhale and touch your chin to the collar bone by bending forward. Repeat 5 times (cervical patients should not bring the chin downward) (Fig. 13.3a).

3. Turn your neck while exhaling towards the right side. Return to original position and inhale. Now turn the neck to the left side in the same manner. Repeat this 5 times (Fig. 13.3b).

4. Bend your neck alternately to both sides, and try to touch the ears to the left and right shoulders (3 to 5 times) (Fig. 13.3c).

5. Rotate the neck in a circular manner starting with the chin touching the chest with eyes closed (clockwise and anti-clockwise simultaneously).

6. Repeat the exercise 2 to 4 times.

- **For ears (Fig. 13.4 a, b, c)**

Position : Stand at ease.

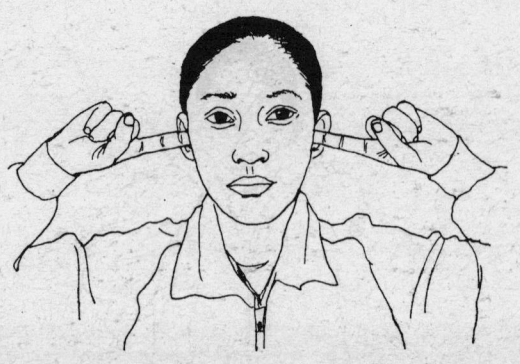

Fig. 13.4b Exercise for ears

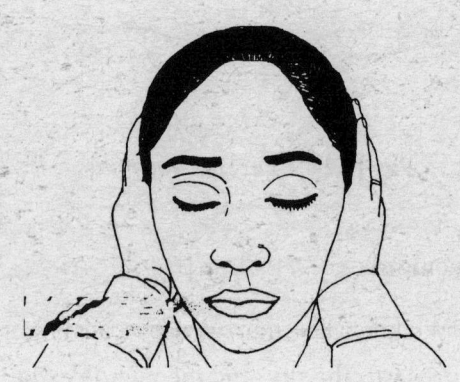

Fig.13.4c Exercise for ears

Movements :

1. Pull up both ears with your hands (5 times) and then pull down the ear lobes (5 times) (Fig. 13.4a).

2. Insert your index fingers in both ears and rotate softly (4 to 5 times) (Fig. 13.4b).

3. Rub and warm up your palms. Cover the whole ear with your palm, press and listen

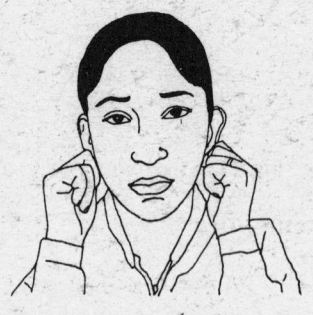

Fig. 13.4a Exercise for ears

Innovative Yogic Life-style Intervention Programme

the inner sound for some time (eyes closed) (Fig. 13.4c).

- **For face**

Position : Stand at ease.

Movements :

1. Rub your face from below upwards using both the palms (5 to 10 times).
2. Feel relaxed and activated.

- **For shoulders (Fig. 13.5 a, b)**

Position : Stand at ease.

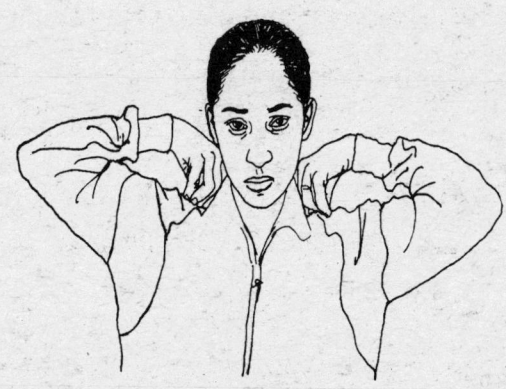

Fig. 13.5 b Exercise for shoulders

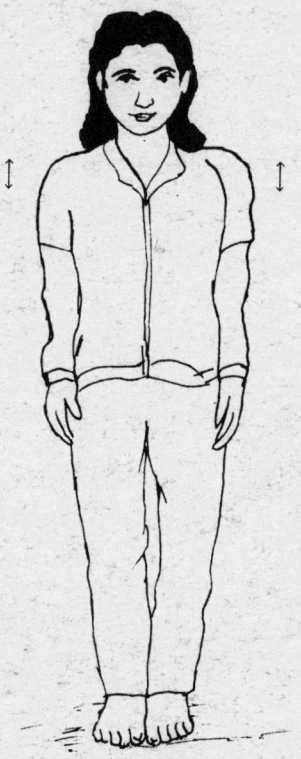

Fig, 13.5a Exercise for shoulders

Movements :

1. Keep your arms hanging straight with semi-closed fists. Raise the shoulders up while inhaling and bring them down while exhaling without bending the elbows (5 to 10 times) (Fig. 13.5 a).

2. Rotate the shoulders from backward to forward, keeping the arms relaxed and also repeat it from forward to backward (5 to 10 times).

3. Bend both your arms with fingers and thumb together at the shoulders. Inhale and rotate the shoulders from forward to backward and then backward to forward (5 times) (Fig. 13.5 b).

Yogic Cure to Avoid Heart Surgery

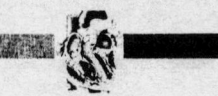

- **For chest and lungs (Fig. 13. 6 a, b)**

Position : Stand at ease.

Movements :

1. Bend both arms, touching palms to the chest, middle fingers of both the hands facing and meeting each other at the middle of the chest.

2. Inhale and extend the left hand, exhale and bring back the hand to its basic position. Repeat the exercise with the right hand also (5 times each).

3. Now do it with both the hands (5 times).

4. Try to inhale and exhale to your maximum capacity, as much as you can do easily.

- **For waist (Fig. 13.7 a, b, c)**

Position : Stand at ease, keep feet apart by your shoulder width, hand at the side of the body

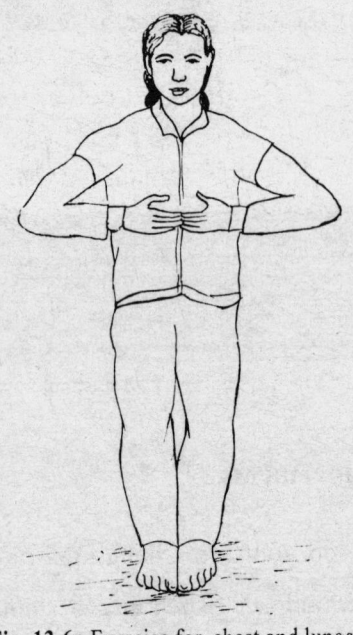

Fig. 13.6a Exercise for chest and lungs

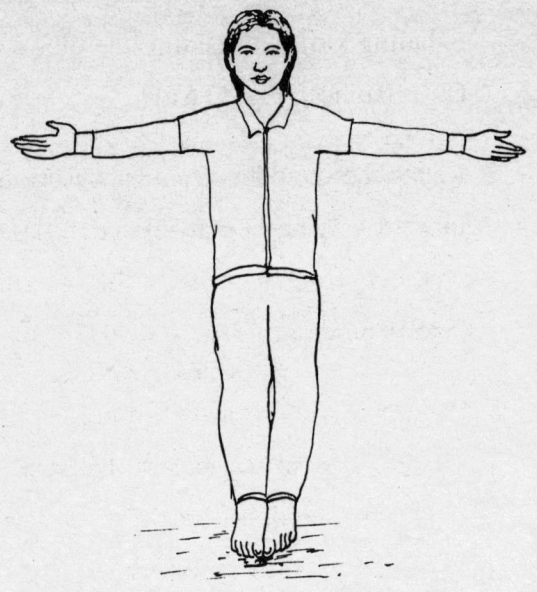

Fig. 13.6b Exercise for chest and lungs

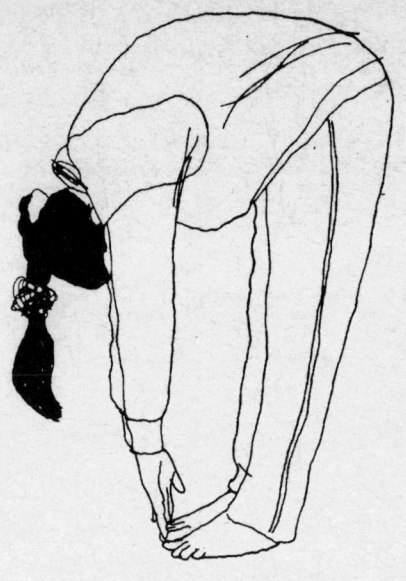

Fig. 13.7a Exercise for waist

Innovative Yogic Life-style Intervention Programme

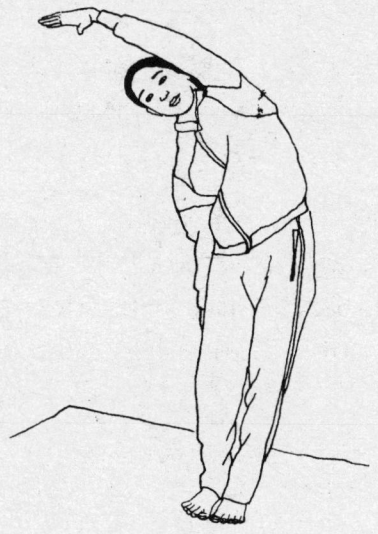

Fig. 13.7b Exercise for waist

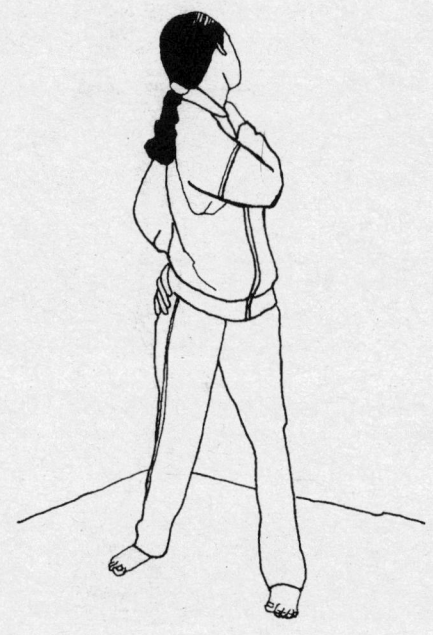

Fig. 13.7c Exercise for waist

Movements :

1. Inhale fully, stretch the hands upwards, move the abdomen forward and shoulders backward and look at the sky. Now exhale and bend forward and try to touch the knees by the forehead, while touching the feet with your hands. Do not force the body, perform the exercise in a relaxed manner. Practice will make it easy (Fig. 13.7 a).

2. Raise hands while inhaling, bend at the waist, about 30° to the left while exhaling, bring the left hand near the knee, bend the neck to the left, stretch the right hand also over the head, maintain for a minute or a half and then come to the normal posture. Repeat this on the right side also (Fig. 13.7 b).

3.a. Lock the fingers and raise the hands, turning the palms towards the sky. Bend at the waist, 30° or more towards the left.

   b. Keep both arms straight, touching the ears. Maintain for a minute or half and return to the position 'a'.

   c. Repeat the exercise towards the right side also (3 rounds).

4.a. Inhale, raise the arms in front of the chest at shoulder level, apart by the chest width, keeping the palms facing each other.

   b. Twist the waist towards the left side, putting the right hand on the left shoulder and the left hand on the right hip from the back side. Maintain the posture for some time, i.e. inhale and exhale 5 to 8 times.

Yogic Cure to Avoid Heart Surgery

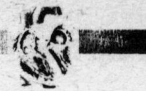

c. Inhale and come to position 'a'.
d. Exhale and bring the hands down.
e. Perform the exercise on the left side also.
f. Please note that almost the whole body would be twisted, but the feet would remain fixed on the floor. (Fig. 13.7 c).

Repeat all exercises 5 times.

- **For thighs and hips**

Position : Stand straight, keeping the legs apart by about 15-20 cm.

Movements :

Strike the buttocks with the heels of left leg and right leg alternately.

- **For feet, knees, ankles, toes and heels** (Fig 13.8 a, b, c, d, e)

Position : Stand at ease but straight, keeping the feet apart by about 15-20 cm.

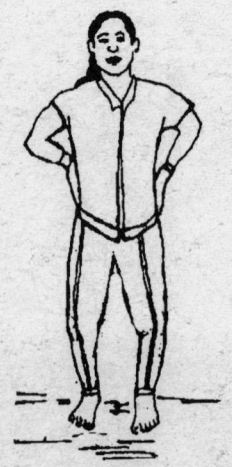

Fig. 13.8b Exercise for feet, knees, ankles, toes and heels

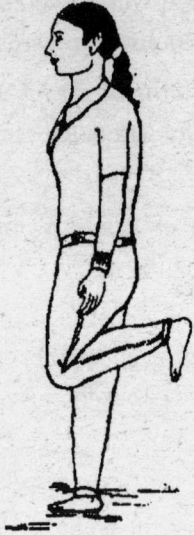

Fig. 13.8a Exercise for feet, knees, ankles, toes and heels

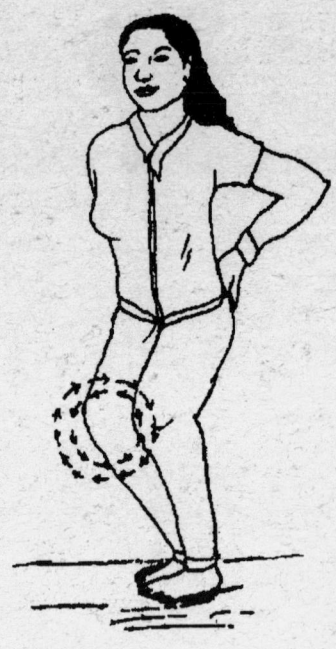

Fig. 13.8c Exercise for feet, knees, ankles, toes and heels

Innovative Yogic Life-style Intervention Programme

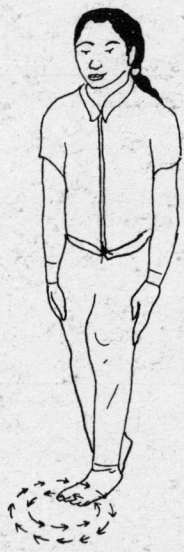

Fig. 13.8d Exercise for feet, knees, ankles, toes and heels

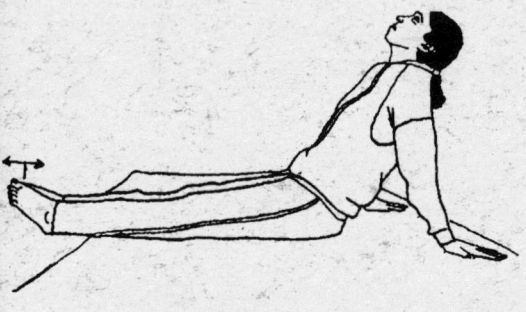

Fig. 13.8e Exercise for feet, knees, ankles, toes and heels

Movements :

1. Let your left heel hit the hip, then stretch foward, feeling a jerk at the knee. Do it with the right leg also. Repeat 5 times (Fig. 13.8 a).

2. Place your hands on the waist, keeping the thumbs in front. Maintain a distance of about 30 cm between the feet. Keep the body straight and bend from knees as low as possible, then come up. Repeat it 5 to 10 times (Fig. 13.8 b).

3. Keep standing with both the feet together. Bend the knees with the palms on waist. Now rotate the knees clockwise and anti-clockwise (5 to 10 rounds) (Fig. 13.8 c).

4. Raise the left leg forward, a little above the ground, with the knees straight. Move the ankle upward and downward 5-6 times. Then rotate at the ankle clockwise and anti-clockwise. Repeat the exercise with the right leg also (5 rounds each) (Fig. 13.8 d).

5. Assume the sitting posture with legs stretched in front of the body (Fig. 13.8 e).

6. Draw the hands in the back of body by the side of the trunk.

7. Lean a little towards the backside with the support of straight arms.

8. Move the toes of both feet slowly backward and forward, keeping the feet stationary (10 times).

9. Now move both feet forward and backward, bending them from the ankle joint (10 times).

10. Now rotate the right and left feet simultaneously around the ankle, both in clockwise and anti-clockwise directions (10 times each).

Yogic Cure to Avoid Heart Surgery

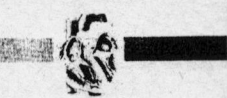

11. Stand erect on your toes, maintain posture for a while, then stand on heels and maintain (5 to 10 rounds).

12. Walk forward on your toes, then backwards on your heels (5 rounds).

Kayotsarga

1. Stand erect or lie down at ease in the sleeping posture with a distance of 30 cm between the legs. Relax your limbs and muscles. Eyes softly closed.

2. Concentrate and spread your mind throughout the body, with a sense of relief from all tensions.

3. Maintain full awareness with slow, deep and long breathing.

4. Feel that your psyche is awakened and body asleep (Fig. 13.9).

5. Do it for 5 to 10 minutes.

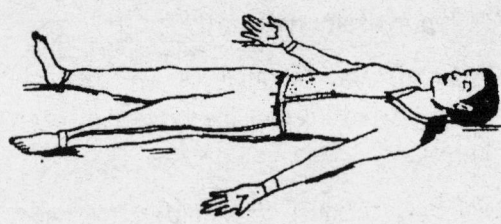

Fig. 13.9 Performance of Kayotsarga

Yogic Asanas

Asanas are a very important component for the yogic intervention in the treatment of CHD. Before you start to perfom asanas, your mind should be calm and free from all apprehensions. Start the asanas in a cheerful state of mind, in an airy and calm atmosphere.

- **Tadasana**

Position : Stand erect, keeping heels and toes parallel and 10 cm apart, or the heels together and toes apart. Arms by the side.

Movements :

1. Raise the arms up with fingers locked, expanding the chest and adbomen slowly. Inhale to the maximum capacity.

2. Raise the body on the toes and hold the posture for sometime, looking at a point at eye level.

3. Keep the knees straight, bring the heels and arms down while exhaling and come to the starting position.

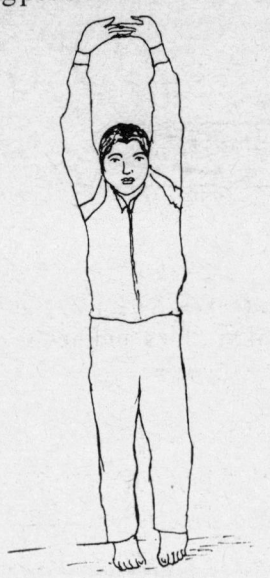

Fig. 13.10 Tadasana

Innovative Yogic Life-style Intervention Programme

- **Padahastasana**

Position : Stand erect with the feet together.

Movements :

1. Raise the arms with palms facing forward over the head while inhaling.
2. Bend forward slowly while exhaling.
3. Bring the palms down to touch the ankles and forehead to the knees.
4. Try to keep the ankles and knees straight.

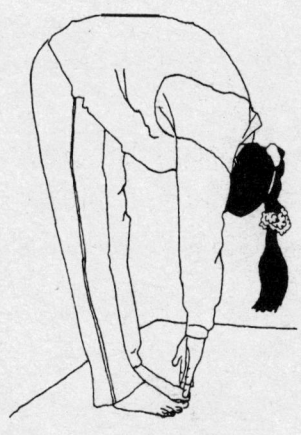

Fig. 13.11 Padahastasana

5. Raise your body upwards slowly while inhaling and taking the arms up.
6. Exhale and bring the arms down.
7. It does not matter if your forehead does not touch your knees, perfectness will be achieved gradually by practice.

Caution :

Any person having slip disc, cervical pain or spondylosis should not practice this asana.

- **Vajrasana**

Position : Kneel down and sit calmly, keeping the waist and neck straight.

Movements :

1. Assume a kneeling position, heels open, toes together facing each other, soles upward.
2. Sit on the soles, keeping the knees together with palms thereon.

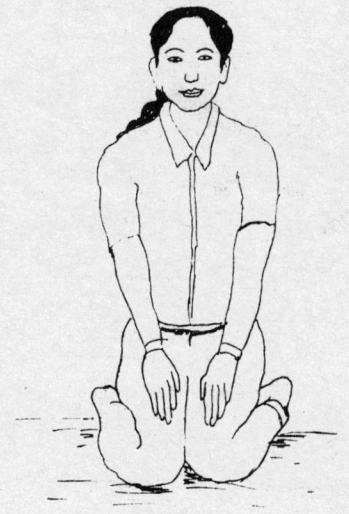

Fig. 13.12 Vajrasana

3. Inhale and exhale slowly and rhythmically.
4. Maintain the posture for some time.

- **Sashankasana**

Position : Sit in Vajrasana with the heels upwards, puting the palms together on knees, keeping the arms straight. The palms should be kept facing each other.

Yogic Cure to Avoid Heart Surgery

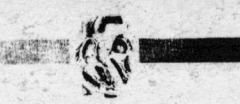

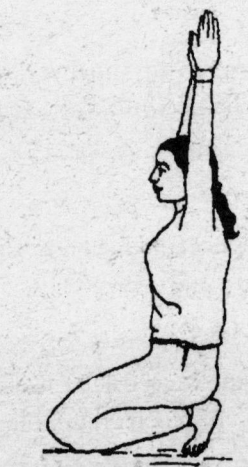

5. Exhale and bring the hands down.
6. Do it twice.

- **Ardhchandrasana**

Position : Stand erect with heels together.

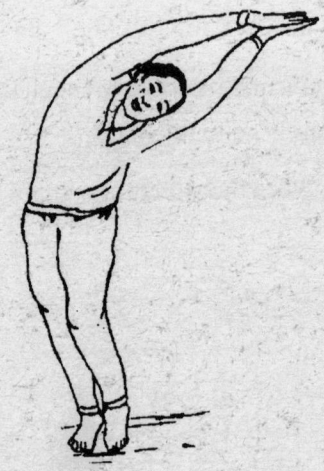

Fig. 13.14 Ardhchandrasana

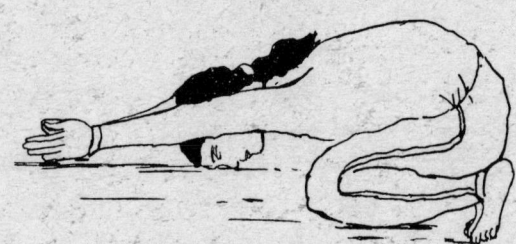

Fig. 13.13 Sashankasana

Movements :

1. Inhale and raise the joined arms over the head.
2. Exhale and bend forward, forehead touching the floor with the palms together.
3. Inhale and exhale peacefully and maintain the posture for 5-10 breaths or more.
4. Inhale and raise the arms along with the head.

Movements :

1. Raise the hands above your head and join them in Namaskar posture.
2. Inhale and bend towards the left from the waist.
3. Exhale and bring the body back in the straight position.
4. Repeat the posture on the right side also.

- **Ardhmatsyendrasana**

Position : Sit on the floor with the legs stretched straight in front.

Innovative Yogic Life-style Intervention Programme

- **Uttanpadasana**

Position (1) : Lie down on the back, keeping the arms parallel to the body and palms towards the floor. Keep the feet together.

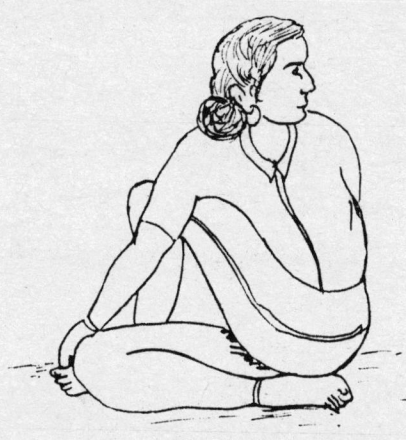

Fig. 13.15 Ardhmatsyendrasana

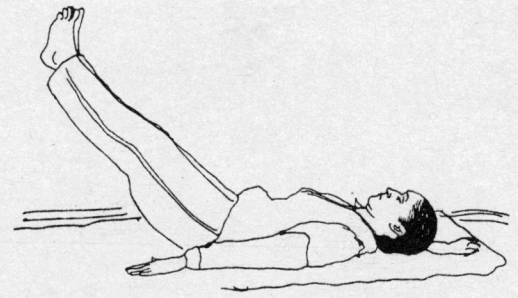

Fig. 13.16 Uttanpadasana

Movements :

1. Raise the right leg, bending a little, the knee upwards and the sole on the floor.
2. Bend the left leg, letting the left heel touch the right hip.
3. Put the right leg and foot by the outer side of the left knee and the right sole on the foor.
4. Bring the left arm-pit over the right knee and hold the right ankle with the left hand.
5. Exhale and stretch the right arm and swing back try to bring it towards the navel.
6. Breathe evenly and maintain this posture for about half a minute.
7. Inhale and bring the right arm to the right side.
8. Exhale and free the left hand and legs.
9. Repeat the posture on the other side too.

Movements :

Position (1):

1. Inhale and exhale. Raise both the legs 15 cm above the floor.
2. While maintaining this posture, inhale and exhale 5 times.
3. Inhale and bring the legs down and exhale.
4. Relax.

Position (2): As per position 1 but keep the legs 30 cm apart.

Movements :

1. Do the same set of movements.
2. Relax.

Position (3): Similar to position 1, but keep the legs 45 cm apart.

Movements :

1. Do the same set of movements.
2. Relax.

Yogic Cure to Avoid Heart Surgery

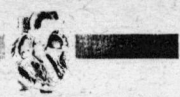

- **Merudandasana**

Position (1) : Lie down in the supine position with the arms stretched at right angles to the trunk.

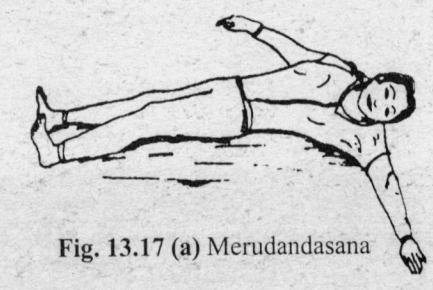

Fig. 13.17 (a) Merudandasana

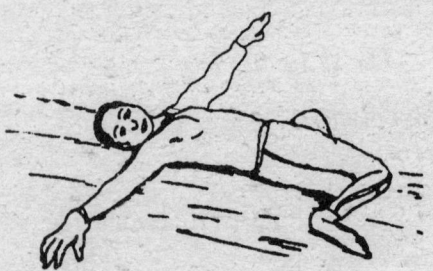

Fig. 13.17 (b) Merudandasana

Movements :

1. Lift the left heel and put it on the right foot between the space of big toe and the second toe, thus keeping the feet straight one above the other.

2. Now stretch and rotate the upper part of the body (head and neck) towards the left and lower parts (waist, thighs and feet) towards the right while inhaling. The left toe should now touch the ground and the arms and shoulders should remain in the same position as before.

3. Come back to the original position while exhaling.

4. Now repeat the same asana on the other side also (5 rounds).

Position (2): Lie down on the back, with the arms stretched at right angles to the trunk.

Movements :

1. Lift the feet with the knees bent apart by about a feet and soles apart by about a couple of feet touching the ground.

2. Now stretch and rotate the upper part of the body (head and neck) towards the left and the lower part (waist, thighs and feet) towards the right side while inhaling. The left knee now should touch the ground and the arms and shoulders remain standstill.

3. Now come back to the original position while exhaling.

4. Repeat the same asana on the other side also (5 rounds).

- **Bhujangasana**

Position (1) : Lie down with face and chest downwards, keeping the heels and toes together. Place the hands near the body, palms towards the floor and forehead touching the ground.

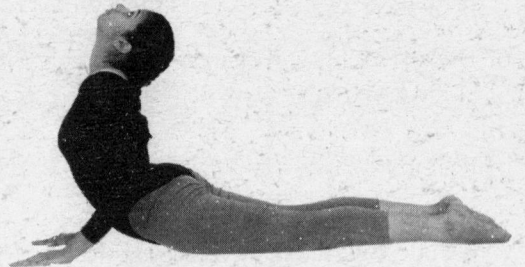

Fig. 13.18 Bhujangasana

Innovative Yogic Life-style Intervention Programme

Movements :

1. Raise the neck about 15cm from the floor while inhaling, and the eyes in front. Raise the trunk a little more. The navel should touch the floor. Maintain this posture for a while.
2. Exhale with a hissing sound and bring the trunk down on the floor. Chin should touch the ground.
3. Take one or two normal breaths.

Position (2) : Bring the hands near the body at a distance of 15 cm.

Movements :

1. Raise your neck 30 cm aboce. Rest of the movements as per position 1.

Position (3) : Now bring the hands near the body at a distance of 30 cm.

Movements :

1. Raise your neck, chest and trunk upwards while inhaling and eyes in front, as much as you can. Arms are straight and erect.
2. Inhale and raise the trunk a little more, body weight should be on the palms and thighs, and look towards the sky. Maintain for some time, giving maximum curve to your chest and abdomen.
3. Exhale slowly with a hissing sound, pulling the nevel inside, and bring the trunk down on the floor.
4. Relax completely for some time, breathe normally, preferably in Shavasana or Kayotsarga.

- **Shalabhasana**

Position : Lie down on your chest, chin touching the floor with arms parallel to the body and palms touching the ground. Legs together, join the heels and put the feet on ground.

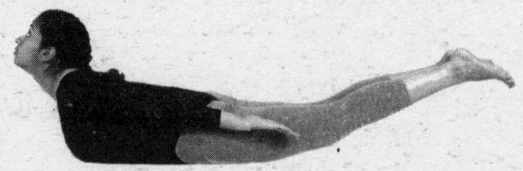

Fig. 13.19 Shalabhasana

Movements :

1. Now place your hands under your thighs; palms sticking to the thighs.
2. Make your body stiff and raise the legs up from the floor as high as you can while inhaling.
3. Hold the posture for some time with normal 2-3 breaths. Do not bend your legs, however, if convinient, raise your face from the ground.
4. Now come back slowly, exhaling, taking the hands out and relax for some time.

Yogic Cure to Avoid Heart Surgery

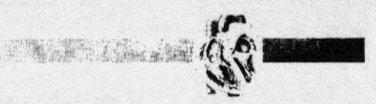

- **Pawanmuktasana**

Position : Lie down on the back, keeping the arms along side the body.

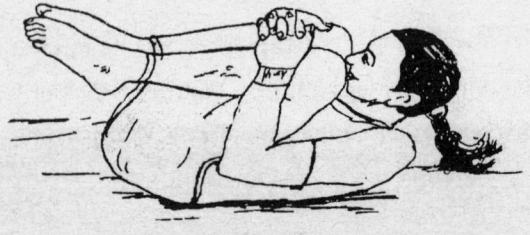

Fig. 13.20 Pawanmuktasana

Movements :

1. Stretch both the legs.
2. Leaving the left leg on the ground, bend the right leg at knee and bring the knee near the chest.
3. Now inhale and press the bent leg on the chest, with both the arms and fingers duly locked.
4. Now take a full breath in the abdomen and go on pressing the leg on it.
5. Now, while exhaling, lift the head and try to touch the nose or the chin with the bent right knee. Maintain for a while.
6. Inhale and bring the head back in the normal position. Also bring the leg down and exhale.
7. Repeat this process with the other leg.
8. Repeat this process with both the legs together.
9. Relax for some time preferably in kayotsarga.

General conditions for performing asanas

Place : Even level, clean, airy and peaceful, preferably outdoors, in an uncrowded garden or warm, ventilated room with an even floor.

Time : Ideally empty stomach in the morning, before dawn, after evacuation of bowels and bladder.

Mattress : Yoga mat, carpet, dari or blanket, but not slippery or too uneven or rough. Thick bed, foam or cushion not appropriate.

Clothes : Loose and limited; avoid belts, pants and other tight clothes.

Duration : 15 to 30 minutes daily. Start with 5-10 minutes, increase gradually.

Benefits of asanas

1. Lack of physical activity is compensated; stiffness in the body organs (a big cause of CHD) is lessened. Foremost positive effect on heart functioning, and facilitating the opening of blocked arteries.
2. Greater oxygenation, lungs are strengthened, heart function and blood circulation are activated, purification is improved.
3. Vertebral column strengthened.

4. Obesity reduced; tension and fatigue reduced.
5. All systemic functions improved and strengthened.
6. Muscles get relaxed, toned, well co-ordinated and improved, efficiency of the functioning of neuro-muscular and skeleto-muscular junctions is improved.
7. Hormonal mechanism improved, secretions of hormones regulated.
8. Restoration and balancing of inner harmony. Negative attitude converted into positive. State of consciousness becomes passive.
9. Ego, fear, anger etc. disappear. Love, affection, satisfaction, happiness and bliss take their place.

Precautions for asanas

1. Always try to perfom yogic exercises and asanas correctly.
2. Know your limits, do not exceed. Increase the duration gradually, even after break of a few days.
3. Be slow and uniform in movements, no jerks allowed.
4. When tired, take rest in between, preferably in the pose of Shavasana.
5. Always use counter postures. If you bend left-ward, right-ward bending is essential.
6. Be regular. Avoid practice during fever/injury.
7. Do not take water immediately after asanas/exercises.

Pranayama (Breathing Exercise)

Introduction : Pranayama is one of the most important components of Patanjali's ashtang yoga. 'Pran' is the vital energy that prevails in each and every element of the universe. 'Pran' does not mean air, but an energy, in muscles it is muscular energy and in the seminal fluid it is sexual energy. The aim of pranayama is to inspire, regulate and balance the 'Pran' shakti in the body. Manu says, *'Just as impurities of gold are removed with the flame of fire, similarly the indriyas (the sense organs) throw their impurities through pranayama'.*

Pranayama is an exercise of breathing; systematic and disciplined breathing. Bathing pures our body, pranayama leads to soundness of mind and body both, strengthening all systemic functions, regulating secretions of hormones and controlling sense organs and **'mana'**. This is the path towards the real knowledge and the real truth.

Technique

Place : Even, clean, airy and peaceful, preferably outdoors and an uncrowded garden.

Time : Ideally, empty stomach in the morning before dawn.

Posture : Padmasana, Vajrasana or Sukhasana. Body erect but not stiff. Hands resting on respective knees, eyes softly closed, in a tense free and cheerful mood.

Yogic Cure to Avoid Heart Surgery

Abdominal breathing

Breath is life. The life begins with the first breath and ends with last.

Abdominal breathing enjoys prominent position in stress management. The practice of abdominal breathing is almost forgotten by the time we grow out of childhood. An infant breathes only abdominally. Of late, advantages of abdominal breathing have been understood very clearly. It at once calms the sympathetic nervous system and activates the parasympathetic nervous system, reducing the heart rate, systolic blood pressure and the oxygen requirment of the heart. In short, it acts like beta-blockers without any side-effects.

Abdominal breathing requires some practice. However, it is very simple and easy to practice in almost any situation. Once the technique is mastered, one may practice it daily under convenient situation, at least 3-4 times a day, for 10-15 breaths each time.

Natural, accurate or abdominal breathing exercise revitalizes our emotinal health, the nervous system and the memory. Its practice not only purifies sinus, cleans nasal passages, lungs and the whole respiratory system, but also improves digestive functioning and relieves constipation. It strengthens the body and spirit both. The breathing exercise may be practiced at times when you are in a relaxed mood, but not to do after meals.

Procedure

1. Lie down on a mat facing your back to the floor. If you feel any discomfort in waist or breathing, bend your knees. Keep your feets apart from hips and the knees resting against each other.

2. Focus your attention on naval area. Place both your hands on belly, palms facing downwards over belly button. Eyes softly closed.

3. Inhale slowly and deeply through your nose keeping the mouth closed and hands fully loose. Feel and immagine that your belly is expanding upwards as if a balloon is inflating. Pause a while.

4. Now exhale slowly and fully through mouth with a ..*hiss*.. sound. Immagine that your belly balloon is deflating and sinking towards your spine. Pause a couple of seconds. Press the belly gently with hands put thereon.

5. Do this exercise for 5 to 10 minutes daily. This will enhance the total duration provided for the gaseous exchange i.e. intake of maximum of oxygen and excretion of carbondioxide to purify the blood. This will also keep you fit, fine and energetic the whole day.

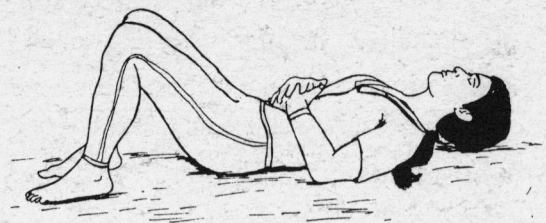

Fig.13.21 Performance of abdominal breathing exercise

- **Anulom-vilom pranayama**
1. Sit in any comfortable posture, keeping the fingers as shown in the picture.
2. Close you right nostril with your right thumb and inhale slowly through the left nostril.
3. When the inhalation is complete, hold the breath for about a second.

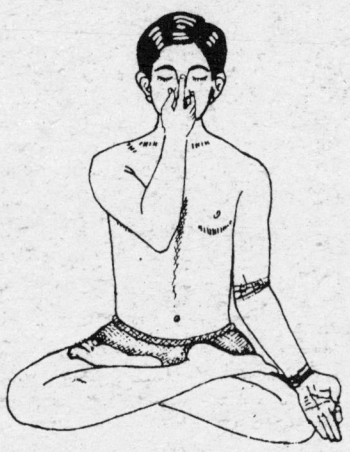

Fig. 13.22 Performance of Pranayama

4. Now lift the thumb from the right nostril, close the left nostril with the finger and exhale slowly through the right nostril.
5. Repeat the process by inhaling through the right nostril and exhaling through the left one.
6. This is one cycle of Anulom-vilom pranayama. Repeat 10 to 20 cycles. Increase the frequency and duration slowly.

- **Om dhwani and laughter**

Om dhwani :
1. Sit in Padmasanaa or Sukhasana, breathe in normally, a bit longer.
2. Say 'O' with a sweet sound, keeping the lips open.
3. Now close the mouth and pronounce 'M' through the nostrils, producing vibration sound like buzzing of a bee. Try to lengthen the sound as much as possible.
4. This is *nad-yoga*, which gives peace of mind, increases concentration power and influences *sushumna* (spinal cord). Will power is developed.

Laughter :
1. Laughing with mouth closed : Laugh internally without a sound. Feel every part of the body smiling.
2. Laughing with mouth open : Laugh with a sound. Feel each part of the body laughing.
3. Laughing loudly : Laugh as loudly as possible and feel your whole body getting energised.

Benefits of Pranayama
1. Pran (vital energy) is amplified. Soul/psyche (chitta) is purified.
2. Act of respiration is prolonged, which strengthens the function of lungs. More oxygenated and purified blood goes to body tissues.
3. Respiratory cycle becomes rhythmic. Lower lobes of lungs become activated, which help in the act of gaseous exchange, i.e. exhange of oxygen and carbon dioxide.
4. Cleaning of nasal passages and opening of eustachian tube is activated.

5. Pranayama, besides strengthening the respiratory system, helps in regulating the blood circulation, nervous system, secretion of hormones and digestion.

6. Favourable effect on heart. Helpful in opening the blocked arteries.

7. General power of resistance increases. Immune system strengthens.

8. Useful in controlling the activity of senses and fluctuation of mind.

9. Above all, the foremost factor is that it helps control stress, the biggest cause of CAD.

Precautions for Pranayama

1. Relax your body and keep your mind calm before commencing pranayama.

2. Know your limits, never exceed.

3. Remember to contract your abdomen while exhaling and to expand it while inhaling.

4. Heart patients to avoid holding of breath.

5. Practice pranayama twice a day, in the morning and in the evening. For better results, concentration on breathing is essential.

6. Never practice pranayama immediately after a bath, breakfast, lunch and dinner.

7. Always practice pranayama in open air, never in bed with the mouth covered.

8. Never practice pranayama in a smoky, dusty atmosphere.

9. Do not drink water immediately after perfoming pranayama (for at least 5 minutes).

Mudras

Mudras also help in the treatment of various diseases. The following two mudras are highly effective in the cure of coronary ailments and lowering high blood pressure. Apan mudra sometimes shows an immediate effect like Sorbitrate, that is why it is called 'Mritjivani mudra'. It normalises the pulse rate also. Vyan mudra is practiced for reducing the high blood pressure.

- **Apan Mudra**

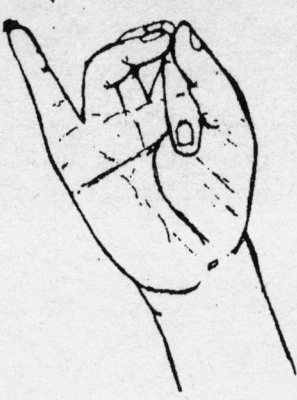

Fig. 13.23 Performance of Apan Mudra

Method : Bend the fore finger to touch the base of the thumb and join the tips of middle finger and ring finger with the tip of thumb.

Innovative Yogic Life-style Intervention Programme

- **Vyan Mudra**

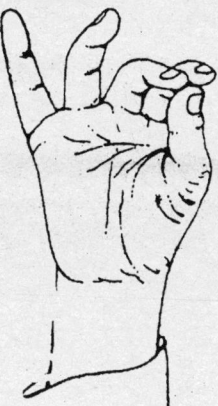

Fig. 13.24 Performance of Vyan Mudra

Method : Join the tip of fore finger and middle finger to the tip of the thumb.

- ### Kayotsarga
  (Total Relaxation with Self-awareness)

Kayotsarga is also a very important wing of yoga/meditation. The literal meaning of kayotsarga is to drop the body. `Kaya'` means body and `utsarg'` means to drop (to experience the detachment of self from body). Kayotsarga has two implications : first, relaxation of mind and body with the awareness of psyche. Second, the existence of two separate identities of body and soul, i.e. body and soul are not one but two; however, they are complementary to each other.

Kayotsarga is a process of autosuggestion. We direct and suggest each and every part of our body including the brain to relax. Then we feel that they are being relaxed. In this process our body and brain sleep, while our psyche remains fully alert. This results in relaxation of muscles and reduction in basal metabolic activities. Consequently consumption of energy in the cells/tissues is reduced and is thus saved. Kayotsarga is physically more restful than a sleep. This exercise helps a lot in releasing mental tension and proves to be an antidote to psychosomatic ailments resulting from mental tensions.

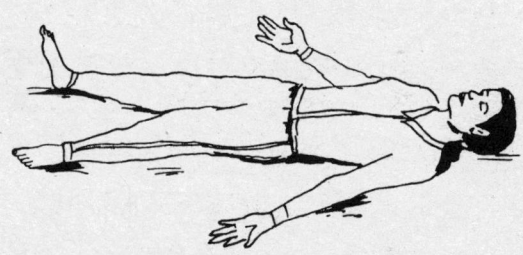

Fig. 13.25 Performance of Kayotsarga

Procedure

Step 1: Perform Tadasana twice or thrice in standing posture.

Step 2: Lie down in supine posture with spine and neck straight, without stiffness, keep 1 feet (30 cm) distance between legs. Hands parallel to the body, palms open skywards. Eyes softly closed.

Step 3 : Keep the body like a statue. No movement at all. Let the whole body become as loose as possible.

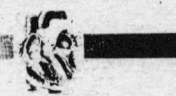

Step 4 : No thinking, no imagination, no memory. Suggest the brain to think 'nothing'. Feel that the body is becoming lighter and lighter.

Step 5 : Now through auto-suggestion focus attention on each and every part of the body from toe to head, one by one, and feel relaxed.

Step 6 : Start relaxation from the right-leg toe, then sole, heel, ankles, calfmuscles, knee, thigh, buttocks and the portions up to the waist. Then in the same way relax the left leg.

Step 7 : Relax the middle part of the body in the same way, i.e. lower abdomen, upper abdomen and organs therein; ribs, chest muscles, shoulders, back-waist, neck and both the hands.

Step 8 : Relax the upper part of the body, i.e. throat, chin, mouth, jaws, tongue, cheeks, nose, eyes, ears, temples, forehead, head-scalp and the brain inside.

Step 9 : Perceive the whole body and experience physical, mental and emotional relaxation. If there is any tension in any part of the body, relax it again and feel that the whole body has become fully relaxed. Maintain this posture for about 15 minutes.

Step 10 : Now imagine that you are sitting on top of mount Everest. You are seeing snow and only snow all around. White clouds are hovering hither and thither by your sides. Feel the sun shining and the atmosphere heavenly, as if you have reached Almighty's home.

Step 11 : Now feel that the whole body has become very light and charged with the Godly energy and vital force.

Step 12 : To complete kayotsarga, take 2-3 deep and long breaths, inhale and exhale, reactivate your body, turn to the left and sit up slowly. Take 2-3 more full breaths.

Precaution : Please do not take water for 5 minutes after kayotsarga.

PREKSHA MEDITATION
(Special Meditation for CHD Patients)

Procedure :

Step 1 : Preparation

(a) Ready for meditation. Adopt the posture you can comfortably sit for about half an hour (30 minutes), i.e. full-lotus, half-lotus, simple crossed legs or the diamond posture.

(b) Adopt 'Brahma mudra', put your hands in the lap, keeping the left palm below the right one, both the thumbs touching each other.

(c) Waist straight, vertebral column straight, eyes softly closed, breathing normal. No tension, cheerful mood. Concentrate in your body only with eyes closed. No thinking, no memory, no imagination.

(d) Maha-pran dhwani : Inhale and produce the sound .. m m m .. through the nostrils like buzzing of a bee. Repeat it 9 times. Try to lengthen and sweeten the echo sound as much as possible.

(e) Say : *'Sam-pikkhae Appaga-mappae-namm'*. 'See your soul through your soul. See thyself by thyself. Know yourself and observe yourself.'

(f) **Sankalp** (pledge) : Say, *'I am practising preksha meditation for purification of my soul, my psyche and to get rid of my heart problem'*.

Repeat the above sankalp thrice.

Step 2 : Kayotsarga (relexation of body and mind)

(a) Please let your whole body loose and relax. Let all the muscles loose and motionless like a statue. No movement at all.

(b) Suggest each and every organ of your body to relax and then feel that they are becoming relaxed...relaxed... relaxed.

(c) Experience the whole body including your brain becoming fully relaxed. Experience relaxation deeper and deeper. Mind should be happy and cheerful.

Step 3 : Shwas preksha (perception of breathing)

(a) Regulate your breathing. Make it slow.

(b) Focus and fix your psyche on your navel and observe its movement. It expands and contracts with every inhalation and exhalation. Try to see only the movement of navel, nothing else.

(c) Now shift your concentration from navel to the juncture of both your nostrils. See and perceive each and every breath going inside and coming outside. Not a single particle of air should move without your knowledge and checking.

(d) Preceive each and every inch of your breath. With perception of breath, we become able to see the truth and God.

(e) Preception of breating is a very good technique for stress release. Stress is the strongest factor for coronary heart disease. Maintain the posture for 5 minutes.

Step 4 : Anupreksha on heart (visualisation of heart)

(a) With your mind's eye, please visualise a green bright light spread around you, a green aura around you, a green pyramid around you. Inhale and exhale green.

(b) Imagine that a green lighted torch bulb is shining upon your thymus gland, i.e. centre of bliss near your heart. This bulb is giving light outside as well as inside, towards your heart. All the four chambers of the heart can clearly be seen in this green light.

(c) Imagine that this green, bright light is penetrating inside your blocked artery, where the blockage has been pointed out by your doctor.

Yogic Cure to Avoid Heart Surgery

(d) Now visualise that the radiation of this green light is reducing your blockage, erasing your blockage, throwing a laser beam on your blockage.

(e) In this situation imagine that a small sticker is affixed near your heart with four lines printed thereon as given under point 'f'.

(f) Read and utter :

(1) Blockage of my artery is being opened.

(2) My heart is becoming cured.

(3) Now there is nothing to worry or fear

(4) Definitely, I will get rid of my heart problem.

Now repeat the above four lines 10-15 times silently.

Step 5 : Jyoti kendra preksha (perception of centre of enlightenment)

(a) Concentrate on Jyoti kendra, the point in the centre of your forehead.

(b) Imagine a white torch-bulb affixed thereon and is spreading white, bright light outside as well as inside the Jyoti kendra. Imagine, as if the full moon has come down and stayed over there.

(c) Now imagine that you are sitting on top of mount Everest in a meditation posture. Snow and only snow is spread everywhere around you.

(d) A huge stock of happiness, bliss and peace is being seen around all the sides. Imagine a white heavenly atmosphere is being showered upon you.

(e) Experience that your aura is being purified and becoming strengthened. Anger, fear, ego and stress have disappeared, and plenty of peace, happiness, bliss, liberty and delight are spreading around you.

(f) Feel, as if you have reached the house of Almighty. You are now able to find the real Truth.

(g) Enjoy this Godly atmosphere for some time. Feel that special vital force and courage has been pumped inside you by the Almightly.

(h) Conclude the meditation session with two or three long breaths.

Step 6 : Follow the stress management

For practice the principles of positive thinking and reflection of moral values, the techniques described in chapters 7 and 8 may be adopted.

Step 7 : Follow the diet management

The details of diet management are given in chapter 12.

CHAPTER 14

Efficacy of Yogic Life-style Intervention Programme in Reversing/Managing CHD (Experimental Research Results)

Contents

14.1	Introduction	153
14.2	Comparative data of CHD patients (before and after yoga therapy)	153
14.3	Discussion and conclusions	160

Efficacy of Yogic Life-style Intervention Programme in Reversing /Managing CHD (Experimental Research Results)

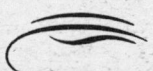

14.1 Introduction

Studies have shown that the modification of risk factors yields positive and favourable effects on the management of coronary heart disease. Dr Dean Ornish had reported that by applying the strategy of `Stress Management' and `Dietary Control', significant beneficial results were obtained in CHD patients. Similarly, Niebaner and Hembrech also showed that a comprehensive life-style change produces significant beneficial effects on CHD patients.

Yogic life-style intervention programme is an effective system of therapy to manage the coronary heart disease even at an advanced stage. It induces reduction in the risk factors, thereby diminishing the occurrence of angina and heart attacks. It successfully helps in reducing the body weight and positively affects the lipid profile and triglycerides, decreasing their levels. It inhibits progression of coronary obstruction and stabilizes other atherosclerotic plaques, reducing the need of revascularisation procedures and leading to blockages. Further, the yogic style of life improves work performance and provides useful and long-lasting strength to the body and mind. It is quite easy to adopt by a heart patient and a common man too because of its very low cost and easy techniques. Moreover, it does not have any side-effects and a practitioner has nothing to lose.

14.2 Comparative Data of CHD Patients (Before and After Yoga Theraphy)

Six patients were examined in one of the camps organised under Yogic Life-style Intervention Programme. Their base line (before treatment) and subsequent development after 3 and 6 months follow- up period in parameters like blood sugar, pulse rate, total cholesterol, LDL and HDL, triglycerides, haemoglobin and subjective mental stress feelings, were recorded. Every individual's comments regarding his/her own feelings were noted along with objective parameters of study.

The comparative data of CHD patients are given here.

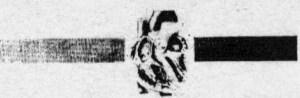

Patient's Progress Chart

Name of patient : Mr `A'`   **Sex :** Male   **Patient no. 1**

Age : 60 years   **Height :** 167 cm (5'.6")   **Marital status :** Married

Profession : Retired government servant

Brief history and general condition before treatment/training

Had a heart attack 6 months back; angiography revealed 100% blockage in one of the coronary arteries; high cholesterol level and hypertension; low HDL; pulse irregular; heaviness and pain in the chest; much depression; had been advised bypass surgery; money deposited for operation.

Changes

Parameter	Before treatment	After 3 months	After 6 months
B.P. (mm of Hg)	160/90	130/85	130/80
Pulse rate	70	70	70
Weight (in kg)	62	60	60
Cholesterol	240	220	200
LDL cholesterol	149	118	112
Triglycerides	140	130	130
HDL cholesterol	20	25	30
Haemoglobin	13	14	15
ST segment depression	3	3	2
Mental stress	Nominal	Nominal	Nominal
Medicine intake	Heavy doses	Sorbitrate reduced	Sorbitrate stopped

Comments of the patient after 6 months of training/treatment

It gives me pleasure to record that yoga and life-style training for CHD treatment has helped me bypass the bypass surgery. My TMT shows improvement. I have stopped taking Sorbitrate tablet. I am highly thankful to my trainers for proper guidance, co-operation and pleasing behaviour during the training. I have now withdrawn my money deposited for the operation. The programme is excellent and the therapy is a miracle. I am away from tension too.

Efficacy of Yogic Life-style Intervention Programme in CHD

Patient's Progress Chart

Name of patient : Mr `B' **Sex :** Male **Patient no. 2**
Age : 56 years **Height :** 170 cm (5'7") **Marital status :** Married
Profession : Sales executive

Brief history and general condition before treatment/training

Old angina patient, smoking habit, using 3-4 Sorbitrate tablets daily. TMT : 7 minutes. Angiography established blockage of 60%, 72% and 90% in all the three arteries. ECG showing higher ST segment depression. Very worried and scared of getting a bypass surgery, as advised. Mentally perturbed.

Changes

Parameter	Before treatment	After 3 months	After 6 months
B.P. (mm of Hg)	130/90	130/85	130/80
Pulse rate	73	73	73
Weight (in kg)	68	66	65
Cholesterol	300	270	240
LDL cholesterol	160	142	139
Triglycerides	200	180	160
HDL cholesterol	20	30	35
Blood glucose (F)	130	125	120
(PP)	180	170	140
Haemoglobin	11	12	12.5
ST segment depression	3	3	2
Mental stress	Highly depessed	Improved a bit	Improved enough
Medicine intake	Heavy doses	Slightly reduced	Considerably reduced

Comments of the patient after 6 months of training/treatment

Immediately after I joined the training (yoga training for CHD treatment), I stopped smoking and never smoked again. Angina problem has now completely disappeared. Sorbitrate tablet is now not needed at all. I joined my duties again after 3 months, when my ECG improved and TMT became normal. I am doing my duties peacefully. Now there is no fear in the mind. My medicine intake is gradually on decline. I now believe that yoga treatment for CHD is the best amongst all present-day therapies, which can avoid very expensive, painful and even risky heart surgery, where re-occurrence of problem is a common feature. Thanks.

Yogic Cure to Avoid Heart Surgery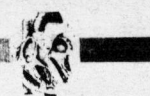

Patient's Progress Chart

Name of patient : Mr 'C' **Sex :** Male **Patient no. 3**
Age : 62 years **Height :** 175 cm (5'9") **Marital status :** Married
Profession : Retired teacher

Brief history and general condition before treatment/training

Heart attack in November 1997. Chest pain; not able to walk even 100 steps. TMT duration 5 minutes. Angiography showed blockages in all three arteries, i.e. 80%, 75% and 85%. Acute depression. Advised angioplasty/bypass surgery.

Changes

Parameter	Before treatment	After 3 months	After 6 months
B.P. (mm of Hg)	160/110	150/110	145/90
Pulse rate	71	71	71
Weight (in kg)	90	86	80
Cholesterol	275	250	220
LDL cholesterol	139	133	118
Triglycerides	150	140	130
HDL cholesterol	20	23	28
Haemoglobin	10	11	12
ST segment depression	3	2	2
Mental stress	Highly depessed	Improved a bit	Improved enough
Medicine intake	Heavy doses	10% reduced	25% reduced

Comments of the patient after 6 months of training/treatment

Before joining the yoga training programme, I could not walk even 100 steps. Now I am able to walk 2 km in the morning and evening. Angina/heaviness in chest is reduced. I feel cured and fit now. Medicines mingled with yoga philosophy of living is crores of rupees worth of prescription for heart patients. Now I do not feel any problem in walking or even in climbing stairs. ECG has improved. The yoga treatment taught me how one can pass a normal life by spending 1 hour a day on yoga, meditation and stress prevention, even after a heart attack.

Patient's Progress Chart

Name of patient : Mr 'D' **Sex :** Female **Patient no. 4**
Age : 50 years **Height :** 157 cm (5'2") **Marital status :** Married
Profession : Housewife

Brief history and general condition before treatment/training

Heart pain, pulse irregular, obese, admitted in hospital for 10 days. Thereafter constant pain in chest. Doctors advised angioplasty. Feeling highly depressed and disheartened.

Changes

Parameter	Before treatment	After 3 months	After 6 months
B.P. (mm of Hg)	160/110	145/110	145/90
Pulse rate	73	73	73
Weight (in kg)	72	69	66
Cholesterol	235	220	210
LDL cholesterol	144	141	127
Triglycerides	200	180	140
HDL cholesterol	25	30	35
Haemoglobin	12	12.5	13
ST segment depression	3	2	1
Mental stress	Depessed	Improved	Improved
Medicine intake	Heavy doses	Reduced	Reduced

Comments of the patient after 6 months of training/treatment

I was highly depressed and had left hope of life. After attending yoga training treatment programme for 10 days, specially `kayotsarga', heart pain was reduced greatly, and I began to feel hopeful towards life. I learnt yoga meditation and value of less-calorie food. After 3 months, my depression was almost over. My weight was reduced by 3 kg within 3 months. I started feeling energetic. Now I hope that with a short span of time more, I will totally become a fit person and my life will be worth enjoying.

Yogic Cure to Avoid Heart Surgery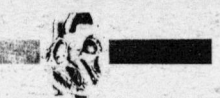

Patient's Progress Chart

Name of patient : Mr 'E' **Sex :** Male **Patient no. 5**
Age : 54 years **Height :** 165 cm (5'5") **Marital status :** Married
Profession : Businessman

Brief history and general condition before treatment/training

Angina. Angiography revealed 90% blockage. Hypertension, diabetic, taking heavy doses of allopathic medicine, overweight; highly depressed. No interest in living. Advised bypass surgery.

Changes

Parameter	Before treatment	After 3 months	After 6 months
B.P. (mm of Hg)	170/100	150/90	145/90
Pulse rate	70	70	70
Weight (in kg)	85	80	75
Cholesterol	250	230	210
LDL cholesterol	152	150	133
HDL cholesterol	25	28	32
Blood glucose (F)	140	130	120
(PP)	180	160	140
Haemoglobin	11	12	12.5
ST segment depression	3	2	2
Mental stress	Highly depressed	Still depressed	Reduced
Medicine intake	Heavy doses	Reduced	Minimised

Comments of the patient after 6 months of training/treatment

After attending the complete training programme, I have achieved a craze for living. My BP and blood sugar have considerably reduced. My weight has been lessened by 10 kg in 6 months. Now I can perform my normal duties well. I have not taken any Sorbitrate tablet during the last 4 months. I feel that not only my heart but all the systems of my body have been activated. Now I can say that if any one follows yogic life-style, there is no need of any hospital or doctor. I am happy and leading a pleasant and normal life.

Patient's Progress Chart

Name of patient : Mr 'F'
Age : 59 years
Profession : Engineer

Sex : Male
Height : 177 cm (5'10")

Patient no. 6
Marital status : Married

Brief history and general condition before treatment/training

In the past I had a sudden heart attack in September 1996 and had gone through angioplasty in October 1996. Still pain and heaviness problem in chest. Cannot walk even 20-30 metres. Breathlessness. Advised bypass surgery.

Changes

Parameter	Before treatment	After 3 months	After 6 months
B.P. (mm of Hg)	130/90	130/90	130/90
Pulse rate	72	72	72
Weight (in kg)	90	87	85
Cholesterol	290	280	260
LDL cholesterol	25	30	35
HDL cholesterol	142	143	139
Haemoglobin	12	13	14
ST segment depression	3	2	1
Mental stress	Highly depressed	Still depressed	Reduced enough
Medicine intake	Heavy doses	Reduced	Reduced

Comments of the patient after 6 months of training/treatment

My general condition after yoga training/practice has improved a lot. Now I can walk around 1 kilometre. Now I neither feel heaviness nor pain in the chest. I am feeling active and fit for performing my regular work/activities as a normal man. My medicine intake has also been considerably reduced. Sorbitrate intake has been totally stopped. Now I am enjoying an angina-free life. Stress management is the most important part of the training/treatment. Diet modification also has its own importance. Love and affection is further very much needed for a CHD patient's life. Exercises/asanas and kayotsarga have impressed me like anything and I am practising the same regularly. I am quite happy and cheeful.

14.3 Discussion and Conclusions

As is evident form the individual subject's record, body weight, lipid profile, triglycerides and blood pressure were found to be reduced uniformly. However, HDL cholesterol level was found increased in all of them. On TMT all the patients were found to be able to exercise for a longer duration and the S.T. segment depression was also found reduced. Mental stress was also reduced and the subjective feeling of well-being was enhanced in all of them. As per their own statements, they felt quite better and energetic.

Coronary arteriography results (which are not produced here due to technical reasons) showed the regression of coronary stenosis in two subjects and it remains unchanged in the rest of the four subjects. This change was again a significant sign of improvement.

In additon, the yoga life-style intervention programme applied to the subjects has not only relieved them from abnormal psychological states, but also reflected no side-effects. Their drug dependency was reduced significantly and they started living a normal, happy life.

On the basis of these findings it can be inferred that yoga life-style programme to manage the CHD has proved quite effective and it may be adopted as an ideal therapy.

Annexures

Contents

1.	Height and weight chart for adults (men/women)	163
2.	Contents of nutrients in some common food items	164
3.	Seven golden rules for CHD prevention	165
(i)	Knowledge about heart functioning and CHD	
(ii)	Knowledge about obesity and hypertension	
(iii)	Knowledge about techniques of stress reduction	
(iv)	Knowledge about diet modification and zero-oil food preparation	
(v)	Knowledge about correct yogic life-style	
(vi)	Knowledge about yogic exercises, asanas and pranayama	
(vii)	Knowledge about meditation and kayotsarga	
4.	Cardio pulmonary resuscitation (CPR)	166
5.	Standard daily routine chart for CHD patients	169
6.	Special benefits of exercises, asanas and pranayama	170
7.	Special benefits of meditation and kayotsarga	170
8.	Emergency stress releasing kit	171
9.	Some clarifications sought by various CHD patients	172
10.	Useful instructions for CHD patients	173

Annexure 1

Ideal Height-Weight Chart for Adults

Height (in cm)	Height (in inches)	Average weight (kg) (for men)	Average weight (kg) (for women)
145	4'9"		46
148	4'10"		46.5
150	4'11"		47.0
152	5'0"		48.5
156	5'1.5"		49.5
158	5'2.2"	55.8	50.4
160	5'3"	57.6	51.3
162	5'3.8"	58.6	52.6
164	5'4.6"	59.6	54.0
166	5'5.4"	60.6	55.4
168	5'6.1"	61.7	56.8
170	5'6.9"	63.5	58.1
172	5'7.7"	65.0	60.0
174	5'8.5"	66.5	61.3
176	5'10"	69.4	64.0
178	5'10.8"	71.0	65.3
182	5'11.6"	72.6	67.0

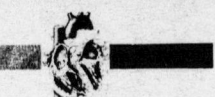

Annexure 2

Contents of Nutrients in Some Common Food Items

(per 100 gm edible portion)

	Name	Moisture	C	P	F	Fibre	Cal.
1.	Rice	13.7	78	7	0.5	0.2	345
2.	Wheat (flour)	12	69	12	1.7	1.9	341
3.	Bengal gram	10	61	17	5.4	1.2	360
4.	Moth bean	11	57	24	1.1	4.5	330
5.	Soybean	8.1	21	43	2.0	3.7	432
6.	Gram	10.4	57	24	1.3	4.1	334
7.	Pea (green)	73	16	7.2	0.1	4.0	93
8.	Green leafy vegetables	90	7.9	2.4	0.7	1.2	30-80
9.	Potato	75	23	1.6	0.1	0.4	97
10.	Carrot	86	11	1	0.2	1.2	48
11.	Radish	94	3.4	0.7	0.1	3.4	17
12.	Sweet potato	69	28	1.2	0.3	0.8	120
13.	Apple	84.6	13.4	0.2	0.5	1.0	59
14.	Cucumber	97	2.5	0.4	0.1	0.4	13
15.	Tomato	93	3.6	1.9	0.1	0.7	23
16.	Banana	70	27.2	1.2	0.3	0.4	116
17.	Guava	82	11.2	0.9	0.3	5.2	51
18.	Grapes	79	16.5	0.5	0.3	3	71
19.	Lemon	85	11	1	1	2	57
20.	Mousmi (orange)	88	9.3	1	0.3	0.5	43
21.	Watermelon	96	3	0.2	0.2	0.2	16
22.	*Muskmelon*	95	4	0.3	0.2	0.4	17
23.	Mutton	71.5	--	18.5	13.3	--	200
24.	Chicken	72	--	26	1	--	109
25.	Cow milk	88	4.4	3.2	4.1	--	67
26.	Skimmed milk	92	5	3	0.1	--	29
27.	Ghee, oil	--	--	--	100	--	900
28.	Sugar	0.4	100	0.1	--	--	400
29.	Honey	21	80	0.3	--	--	320
30.	Egg white (33 gm)	88	0.4	3.4	--	--	16

C = carbohydrate; P = protien; F = fat

Annexure 3
Seven Golden Rules for CHD Prevention

Coronary heart disease obviously is a result of prolonged wrong life-style, lack of physical activity, overweight, excessive cholesterol, excessive stress and wrong food habits. If we are able to gain adequate knowledge of their course and cures, we can definitely keep CHD away. The light of knowledge can easily drive away the darkness of ignorance. Here are some salient rules to follow :

1. Knowledge about heart functioning and CHD : The knowledge about heart functioning and CHD helps us to handle the disease properly to a great extent. But only the knowledge would not be suffcient to serve the purpose; we would have to be practical to achieve the goal.

2. Knowledge about obesity and hypertension : Obesity and hypertension are also the important causing factors of CHD. We should know the techniques of lowering cholesterol levels and reducing high blood pressure.

3. Knowledge about techniques of stress reduction : Stress, though was not recognised as a CHD factor previously, has proved in the recent decades to be one of the biggest causative factors of CHD. Therefore, we must know about its source, manner of its induction and creation, and the technique of its eradication.

4. Knowledge about diet modification and zero-oil food preparation : Since diet plays a very important role to keep one's health in order, wrong food should be dreaded, to be touched only with hot iron tongs. We should learn what is to be eaten, what is to be avoided, and what strictly must not be touched in order to maintain health. Zero-oil food preparation is a healthy habit.

5. Knowldge about correct yogic life-style : The root cause of people's ill health is a wrong life-style. We must know the minus points of modern living, and how they can be modified to keep our body fit. Yoga offers an easy and practical way to maintain and improve one's health.

6. Knowledge about yogic exercises, asanas and pranayama : The modern economic growth and technical developments give a false impulse to the man, not to work and live idle. This tendency has become a symbol of modern advanced society. Consequently the physical activity has become the subject of ancient history. Thus to cope with this deficiency and to face the curse of polluted environment, we should practice yogic exercises, asanas and pranayama.

7. Knowledge about meditation and kayotsarga : The thoughts, attitudes and characteristics of every individual now-a-days are self-centred. He has forgotten the society, morals and God. Therefore in order to maintain his mental peace and inner happiness, the knowledge of meditation and kayotsarga is very essential. These are the powerful tools nto overcome the cynicism and release the stress.

Yogic Cure to Avoid Heart Surgery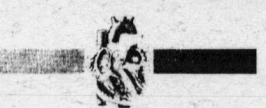

Annexure 4

Cardio-pulmonary Resuscitation

Sudden heart attack : Cardio-pulmonary resuscitation (CPR) acts as an emergency first-aid during heart attack. One of the most startling ideas of modern therapy is that sudden death can be reversed. More astonishing is the fact that this may be achieved by any one of us, using only our lungs and brains. Before sudden death results in final biological death, proper and prompt CPR can revive a person.

The incidences of coronary heart disease are increasing rapidly in India. Around 10% of the people suffering from coronary heart disease die of heart attack every year in India. Out of each 100 people dying of heart disease, 50 die due to heart attack and most of them due to sudden death. About two-thirds of the deaths from heart attack occur before the victim reaches the hospital; out of 24 lakh people dying of heart attack every year, 18 lakhs die before reaching there. An average patient has to wait for nearly 3 hours before medical aid is made available in our country. With the mass CPR programme, around 13.5 lakh people may be saved each year. Remember, sudden-death victims are the ones who count more to the country, i.e. intellectuals and professionals.

CPR cardio-pulmonary resuscitation is administered when a person's pulse or breathing or both stop. Stopping of pulse and breathing is normally called sudden death.

Signals of heart attack : The most common symptoms are uncomfortable breath, squeezing and unbearable pain in the centre of the chest behind the breast bone. One may have a feeling of constriction or as if an elephant is sitting on the chest. Pain may radiate to the left arm, jaw, teeth, left shoulder or less commonly to the right hand or right side of the chest. Other signals may be :

- Unexpected sweating
- Nausea
- Shortness of breath, or
- A feeling of extreme exhaustion or fatigue

Risk factors : Suspect a heart attack at the occurrence of any of the above-mentioned symptoms, especially if the person has the following :

- Diabetes
- High blood pressure
- Elevated cholesterol levels
- Chronic smoker
- Overweight
- Tense/stressful personality
- Family history of heart attack
- Personal history of anginal attack

Precaution : If a person shows any of the symptoms mentioned above, chances are there

Annexures

that he/she has had a heart attack.

Do's

- Make the person lie down flat on the floor or hard bed.
- Raise the legs; this will divert the blood to the brain, and is alone equivalent to giving 2-3 bottles of blood to the person.
- Let fresh air reach the person.
- Start the ABCs of CPR.

Dont's

- Try to make the person sit or stand.
- Put a pillow under the neck.
- Pour water or *Ganga-jal* into the mouth.
- Crowd around the victim.
- Waste time for the doctor to arrive.

ABC's of CPR

A — Airway (wind pipe)

B — Breathing (artificial)

C — Circulation

A. Airway : On opening the airway passage, a person may be saved. Lift up the chin with one hand while pushing down on the forehead with the other hand to tilt the head back. Once the airway is open, place your ear close to the victim's mouth, and

Look — at the movement of the chest

Listen — for breath sounds

Feel — for breaths on your cheek

If no response, i.e. if breathing in the airway does not cause spontaneous breathing, start B.

B. Breathing : The best way to reactivate the breathing process is mouth-to-mouth breathing or mouth-to-nose breathing. It can be done by keeping the head tilted and chin in a lifted position. Pinch the victim's nose and give two full breaths while maintaining an air-tight seal with your mouth on the victim's mouth while giving breaths.

Do's

- Give 2 full breaths at once.
- See for simultaneous chest expansion.
- Give only short breaths.
- Give mouth-to-nose breathing, if mouth-to-mouth is not possible. Close the mouth while giving mouth-to-nose breathing.

Dont's

- Be shy of giving mouth-to-mouth respiration, regardless of the person's sex or age.
- Be afraid of getting a disease or an infection while doing so. (To prevent this, always keep a piece of fine cloth between your and victim's mouth.)

C. Circulation : After 2 full breaths locate the victim's artery, carotid artery or pulse, to see if the heart is beating. To feel a carotid pulse, take your hand that is supporting the chin and locate the Adam's apple (voice box). Slide the tips of your fingers down into the groove beside the Adam's apple and feel for the pulse. If there is no pulse, start cardiac massage with rhythmic pressure on the lower half of the victim's breast

Yogic Cure to Avoid Heart Surgery

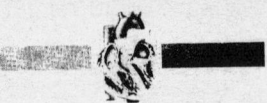

bone; you can force the heart to pump blood.

How to do cardiac massage :

1. Kneel at the victim's side near the chest.

2. With the middle and index fingers of the hand, locate the notch where the bottom rims of the two halves of the rib cage meet in the middle of the chest.

3. Place the heel of one hand on the sternum (breast bone) next to the fingers which meet in the middle of the notch.

4. Place your other hand on top of the one that is in position.

5. Be sure to keep your fingers up, off the chest wall.

6. Interlocking the fingers may help.

7. Bring your shoulders directly over the victim's sternum as you compress downwards.

8. Keeping your arms straight, depress the sternum about 1 to 2 inches (2 to 5 cm) for an adult victim.

9. Then release pressure on the sternum completely.

10. Keep your hand on victim's sternum in between the compressions.

11. Relaxation and compression should be of equal duration.

How long to continue CPR : Continue uninterrupted CPR until advanced life support is provided to the patient.

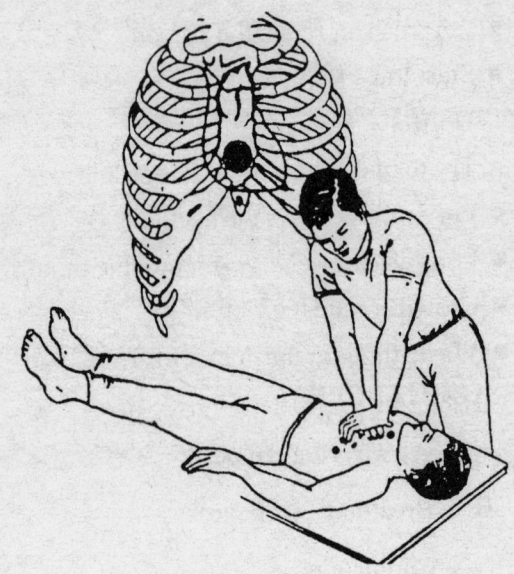

Fig. 15.1 A person performing cardio-pulmonary resuscitation

Annexure 5
Standard Daily Routine Chart for CHD Patients

Time	Component
5.00	Be awake and get up
5.15 to 5.30	Yogic exercises
5.30 to 6.00	Yogic asanas
6.00 to 6.30	Meditation, Kayotsarga, Shwas-preksha, Anupreksha with green colour visualization on heart
6.30 to 7.30	Morning routine
7.30 to 8.00	Breakfast
8.30 to 12.30	Professional routine

Part I

Time	Component
12.30 to 1.00	Kayotsarga
1.00 to 1.30	Lunch
1.30 to 2.30	Rest
2.30 to 4.30	Professional routine

Part II

Time	Component
4.30 to 5.00	Kayotsarga
5.00 to 5.30	Evening walk
5.30 to 6.30	Self-study (swadhyaya)
6.30 to 7.30	Entertainment (T.V., music)
7.30 to 8.00	Meditation
8.15 to 8.45	Dinner
8.45 to 10.00	General work
10.00	Go to bed for a sound sleep

Note : Duration of all components may be adjusted according to convenience and capacity. Regularity and punctuality must be maintained.

Remember : No stress, no anger, no jealousy, no sedentary life, no laziness, no comments on others' lapses.

Try to : Remain happy and cheerful, friendly to all; be contented, peaceful and inwardly strong. Be paticular for: regularty in exercise, asanas, kayotsarga, meditation and walking.

Annexure 6

Special Benefits of Exercises, Asanas and Pranayama

1. Enhancement of physical performance and efficiency.
2. Better control of angina, blood pressure, body weight and fat distribution in the body.
3. Better organ and limb circulation and increase in lung efficiency.
4. Protection of bones and joints, better bowl function and increase of life-span.
5. Enhancement of energy and enthusiasm.
6. Better relaxation and sleep. No sleeping pills/drug required.
7. Better ability to cope with stress, anxiety and depression.
8. Reduction in medical expenses.

Annexure 7

Special Benefits of Meditation and Kayotsarga

1. Better supply of oxygen to lungs.
2. Increase in flexibility and physical fitness.
3. Decrease in hypertension (high blood pressure), pulse rate and heart rate.
4. Reduction in oxygen consumption, anxiety level and serum level.
5. Conversion from Type A personality to Type B personality.
6. Sleeplessness gets subsided.
7. Reversal of CHD.

Annexure 8

Emergency Stress Releasing Kit

In the modern age of technology and so called modern life style, the 'Stress' has become integral problem of every one's life, irrespective of caste, creed, sex and profession. On various singular occasions one has to perform several duties in a stipulated time.

Emergency meetings with senior officers to discuss plan of action without any prior preparation, many household work of a housewife at one time along with guests' hospitality, examination days for students, heavy dues payment for a businessman at a time, commitment of supply orders to be fulfilled for an entrepreneur, and simultaneous health problems within family, are few common examples, where the person concerned comes in such a situation that he or she is not able to decide - how to proceed, what to do first and what latter? How to cope-up with the emergency requirement?

Such situations cause very high degree of stress within the person which ultimately results in utter confusion. Inspite of best capacity one looses the decisive power and efficiency. For such situations the under mentioned 'Emergency Stress Releasing Kit' may be practised to get out of the stressful and tense conditions and to develop stamina of both concentration and right decision.

Procedure

It requires only 4 to 5 minutes performing. When you feel high stress, immediately adopt any meditative posture, sitting or standing with eyes softly closed. Now regulate your breathing and make it slow deep and rhythmic. Focus your concentration on your naval area and observe belly movements. Concentrate on the belly movements and nothing else. At the same time try to inhale and exhale maximum amount of air calmly.

After practicing this process for a couple of minutes only, you will feel yourself more energetic.

Now shift your concentration from naval to the juncture point of your both the nostrils. Just see and perceive each and every breath. Not a single breath should go inside or come outside the nostrils without your knowledge. As a result you will find that all thoughts have been vanished from your brain, which may also be called as thought 'free mind'. However, if you do not reach up to that position, with hold your breath for 2-3 seconds, the thoughts causing confusion and tension will at once disappear. Practice the process for 3 to 4 minutes.

Now open your eyes and return to the work. You will wonder your stress has been reduced to a great extent and now you are feeling to start work afresh with more zeal, stamina and strength.

Yogic Cure to Avoid Heart Surgery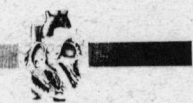

Annexure 9

Some Clarifications Sought by Various CHD Patients

1. People are afraid, with a misunderstanding that the asanas/exercises involve extra exertion, which puts increased load on heart functioning. But in fact, asanas/exercises exert even less load on the heart than walking, because in asanas/exercises some specific parts of the body work and the other parts of the body relax simultaneously, whereas in walking the whole body has to function.

2. Very often is it asked, "Why so many asanas/exercises? Only the asanas directly concerned with the heart should be undertaken, as the asanas put extra load on the heart, which is already sick".

In this regard it may be clarified that the main cause of the blockage in the arteries is the stiffness/hardness of the arteries. When we practice asanas/exercises, the muscles as a whole become flexible, and consequently the arteries too, which is obviously helpful in opening of the blockages occurred in the arteries.

3. The doctors generally advise CHD patients to walk slowly. This is also a very good exercise for them. But remember never to go for a walk immediately after meals, as our energy is diverted and concentrated towards digestive action soon after taking a meal. Hence, there must be a gap of 30-40 minutes. Perform rest for at least half an hour after every meal before you step out.

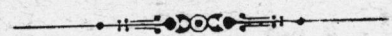

Annexure 10

Useful Instructions for CHD Patients

1. Try to remain physically fit, mentally alert and vigilant, emotionally happy and cheerful.

2. Reduce the stress by :

(a) Adequate planning of your work and time.

(b) Avoiding the postponement of the events.

(c) Sparing time for recreation.

(d) Using specific formula of Do's and Dont's.

   (under chapter 6.3)

3. Try to change and modify the modifiable risk factors.

4. Try to adhere strictly to the planned schedule.

5. Try to perform physical exercise timely and regularly.

6. Try to consume prescribed and balanced vegetarian diet only.

7. Stop smoking completely, if you are a smoker.

8. Try to live in the state of no stress, no anger, no jealousy, no laziness, no sedentary life, no comments on others' lapses.

9. Try to adopt the 'yogic life-style intervention programme' strictly, including kayotsarga (relaxation), meditation, dietary modification, stress management, asanas, exercises, pranayama, laughing and walking, as prescribed in the book.

10. Remain happy and cheerful, friendly to all, inwardly strong and contented with what the Almightly has blessed you, with peace in mind.

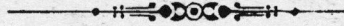